Understanding
Irritable Bowel Syndrome

Dr Kierar

Published by Family Doctor Publications Limited
in association with the British Medical Association

© Family Doctor Publications 2001–2006
Updated 2002, 2003, 2004, 2006

Family Doctor Publications, PO Box 4664, Poole, Dorset BH15 1NN

ISBN: 1 903474 48 5

Contents

About the author

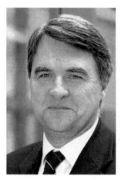

Dr Kieran J. Moriarty, CBE is a Consultant Physician and Gastroenterologist. He has wide experience in the treatment of patients with gastrointestinal disorders. His research interests include abdominal pain, alcohol, IBS and bowel disorders. In 2002 he was awarded the CBE for services to medicine.

Introduction

What is irritable bowel syndrome?

Irritable bowel syndrome (IBS) is one of the most common gastrointestinal disorders, but it is puzzling for those who have it and for the doctors who treat it. Unlike disorders such as stomach ulcers or arthritis, there is no laboratory test, X-ray, scan or endoscopic investigation that can show whether or not you have IBS.

There is no clear-cut cure for the disorder. However, various kinds of treatment can relieve the symptoms and, with the right kind of support from your doctor, you can learn to live with it.

IBS is a syndrome, a collection of symptoms with similar features that occur together in a pattern that your doctor can recognise. In typical cases, there is rarely any doubt about the diagnosis, although you may have symptoms in any part of your gastrointestinal tract, which stretches from the oesophagus (gullet) to the rectum.

What are the main symptoms?

The term 'irritable' is used to describe the reaction of the muscles in the intestine, which respond to stress by abnormal contractions. These may result in various combinations of the three main symptoms:

- pain
- diarrhoea
- constipation.

These symptoms are often worrying. However, if you have been told that you have IBS, you can take some comfort from the information that the disorder does not increase your chance of developing long-term serious conditions such as cancer or ulcerative colitis. Also, there is no evidence that people with IBS have a shorter life expectancy.

What will I find in this book?

The first five chapters of this book describe the structure and working of the gastrointestinal tract. They explain the symptoms of IBS and how it is recognised. They also cover what is known about its causes and how common it is in people from different ethnic groups in countries around the world.

Later chapters deal with common symptoms such as constipation and diarrhoea. They explain how these apparently opposite problems can be part of the same syndrome. These chapters also describe the various approaches to treatment that may be tried and how these can help. There is also practical advice on self-help measures that you may try.

The final chapters of the book discuss how people with IBS can learn to live with the disorder, and get support from a sympathetic doctor. The more that you understand about IBS and the reasons for your symptoms, the better you will be able to cope with them. We hope that this book will help you to do just that.

How common is IBS?

Irritable bowel syndrome affects around one in five adults in the industrialised countries. Even more people have at least one of its symptoms. A study in the USA found that, in one year, as many as 70 per cent of the general population had problems associated with abnormal bowel function, such as abdominal pain, constipation or diarrhoea.

Three-quarters of people with symptoms of IBS do not consult a doctor, and yet as many as half the people seen in a hospital outpatient clinic for gastrointestinal disorders have it as the cause of their problems. Evidence suggests that half the people with IBS seen in clinics also have symptoms of depression or anxiety.

In the UK, around eight million people have IBS. On average, each of them has 17 days off work a year, at an annual cost to the country of £500 million. Average work days missed in the USA per year were 14.8, compared with 8.7 in those without symptoms of IBS. Indeed, IBS ranks close to the common cold as a leading cause for absenteeism from work as a result of illness.

Symptoms of IBS are equally common in men and women, but women consult their doctors about these symptoms more often than men. About half of those with IBS develop symptoms before the age of 35; 40 per cent of people with the condition are aged 35 to 50 years.

There is a tendency for symptoms to occur less often as you get older, but some people do experience them for the first time later in life. Doctors tend to be more cautious about diagnosing IBS in elderly people. They will usually do so only after excluding other diseases of the gut.

KEY POINTS

- IBS is a syndrome, not a disease, affecting about 20 per cent of adults in industrialised countries.

- Doctors see twice as many women as men with the condition

- IBS has a major social impact, leading to frequent days off work and restriction of social activities

The gastrointestinal tract

What is the gastrointestinal tract?

The gastrointestinal tract is a long passageway that connects the mouth and anus. Digestion starts in the mouth, where food mixes with salivary enzymes. When you swallow, food is propelled down the oesophagus (gullet) into the stomach. In the stomach, it is broken down by the powerful digestive enzymes and the hydrochloric acid found in gastric juices.

From the stomach, food passes into the small intestine (duodenum, jejunum and ileum), where juices from the pancreas and gallbladder continue the digestive process. It is here that most nutrients are absorbed from the food. This happens as the intestinal contents are moved along by peristalsis (movement caused by alternating muscle contraction and relaxation).

Undigested waste (faeces) then moves into the large intestine (the colon). In the first part of the colon, muscle contractions slowly move it along towards the rectum while excess water is removed.

The gastrointestinal tract and the digestive process

Food must be broken down so that the body can absorb the nutrients. Undigested material and waste are expelled.

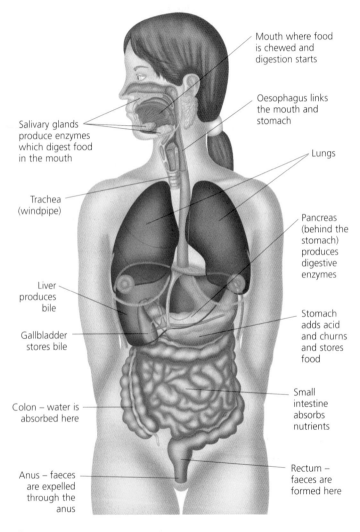

Mouth where food is chewed and digestion starts

Oesophagus links the mouth and stomach

Salivary glands produce enzymes which digest food in the mouth

Lungs

Trachea (windpipe)

Pancreas (behind the stomach) produces digestive enzymes

Liver produces bile

Stomach adds acid and churns and stores food

Gallbladder stores bile

Colon – water is absorbed here

Small intestine absorbs nutrients

Anus – faeces are expelled through the anus

Rectum – faeces are formed here

Just before defecation (bowel action), the waste is moved into the rectum and is then eliminated through the anus.

Daily fluid intake and loss

The intestines are capable of both absorbing and secreting fluid. Overall, it is estimated that nine litres of fluid pass through the intestines each day, of which only around two litres come from food and drink. The other seven litres are secreted by the body itself, in the form of saliva, bile and the juices of the stomach, pancreas and intestine.

These secretions provide the necessary conditions for rapid digestion of nutrients and for optimal absorption of nutrients and minerals. Of the nine litres, approximately 8.8 litres or more are reabsorbed back into the blood, so that less than 200 grams of water are excreted in the stools each day.

The intestines are therefore efficient, reabsorbing as much as 98 per cent or more of the water and minerals that pass through them. If anything prevents this from happening, so that less than 98 per cent of water is reabsorbed, then stool output will be more watery and you will have diarrhoea.

The large intestine

Normally, in the colon, the liquid material entering from the small intestine becomes solid as water is absorbed from it. This solid is then stored until it is convenient for you to open your bowels.

If you are an adult consuming a typical western diet, about 90 per cent of the 1.5 litres or so of liquid reaching your colon in a 24-hour period are absorbed. This leaves 200 millilitres of semi-solid material to be excreted.

The digestive process and daily fluid intake and loss

Liquid is added as digestive juices in the mouth, stomach and duodenum. The intestines both absorb and secrete fluid. Overall, it is estimated that nine litres of fluid pass through the intestines each day. Only around two litres of this comes from food and drink. The other seven litres are secreted by the body itself, in the form of saliva, bile and juices of the stomach, pancreas and intestine. The intestines are very efficient, reabsorbing as much as 98 per cent or more of the water and minerals that pass through them.

Key to diagram on opposite page

——	Oral intake
——	Saliva
——	Bile secretion
——	Gastric juices
——	Pancreatic secretions
——	Intestinal secretions
——	Reabsorption of water in intestines

The daily intake of water and the secretions within the body are efficiently absorbed by the gastrointestinal tract.

Source	Quantity of water
Oral intake	2,000 ml
Salivary glands	1,500 ml
Stomach	2,500 ml
Bile	500 ml
Pancreas	1,500 ml
Intestine	1,000 ml
Total water presented to the intestines	9,000 ml
Expelled in faeces	200 ml
Absorbed by the intestines	8,800 millilitres (ml)

The digestive process and daily fluid intake and loss (contd)

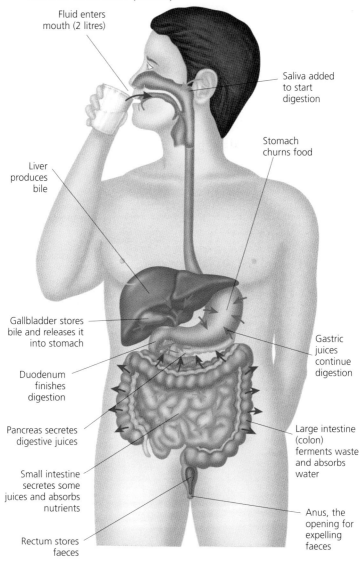

Fluid enters mouth (2 litres)

Saliva added to start digestion

Stomach churns food

Liver produces bile

Gallbladder stores bile and releases it into stomach

Gastric juices continue digestion

Duodenum finishes digestion

Pancreas secretes digestive juices

Large intestine (colon) ferments waste and absorbs water

Small intestine secretes some juices and absorbs nutrients

Anus, the opening for expelling faeces

Rectum stores faeces

The role of the intestines

Partially digested material enters the small intestine from the stomach. Liquid material enters the colon (large intestine) from the small intestine. It progressively solidifies as water is absorbed from it.

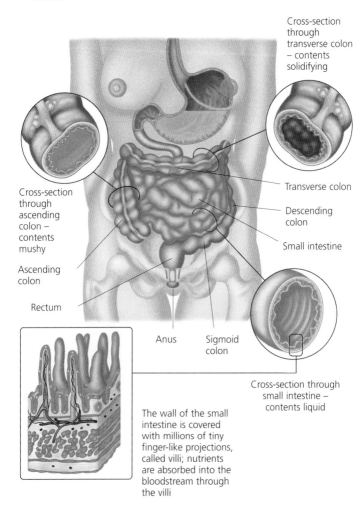

Cross-section through transverse colon – contents solidifying

Transverse colon

Cross-section through ascending colon – contents mushy

Descending colon

Small intestine

Ascending colon

Rectum

Anus

Sigmoid colon

Cross-section through small intestine – contents liquid

The wall of the small intestine is covered with millions of tiny finger-like projections, called villi; nutrients are absorbed into the bloodstream through the villi

Food spends around 1 to 3 hours in the stomach, 2 to 6 hours in the small intestine and 12 to 48 hours in the colon. Normally, it passes through the colon relatively slowly so as to allow fluid to be absorbed. This absorption occurs mainly in the ascending and transverse colon.

Powerful muscle contractions propel solidified stool into the lower (sigmoid) colon and rectum several times a day. Defecation ultimately occurs as a result of complex interactions between sensory and motor nerves within the gut wall and the central nervous system. This interaction stimulates the muscles which empty the rectum. The muscles in the pelvis and rectum contract and the ring of muscle that controls the anus (the anal sphincter) relaxes in a coordinated way.

Transit times through the colon are usually shorter in men than in women, and men's stools are heavier.

Progress of food through the body

After swallowing, food is moved by muscular contractions through the digestive system. The time spent in each part depends on the stage of digestion. It also varies with food type and quantity, and from day to day. The usual total time can vary from 15 hours to 5 days.

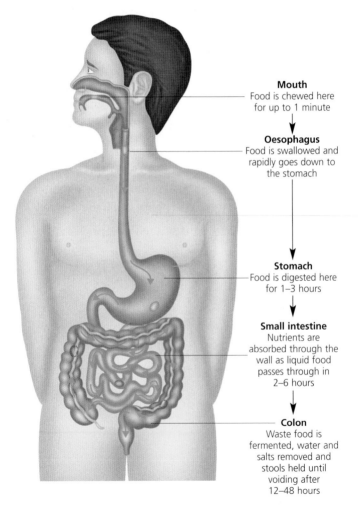

Mouth
Food is chewed here for up to 1 minute

Oesophagus
Food is swallowed and rapidly goes down to the stomach

Stomach
Food is digested here for 1–3 hours

Small intestine
Nutrients are absorbed through the wall as liquid food passes through in 2–6 hours

Colon
Waste food is fermented, water and salts removed and stools held until voiding after 12–48 hours

KEY POINTS

■ The gastrointestinal tract extends from the mouth to the anus; it digests and absorbs food and liquids and propels them along by muscle contraction

■ The small and large intestines are very efficient at absorbing fluid, so that most people excrete no more than 200 millilitres of stools per day; if absorption is impaired by disease, the result is diarrhoea

■ The large intestine consists of the colon, rectum and anus; transit through the colon is slow, which helps absorption of fluid

■ Muscle contractions move solid stool into the lower colon and rectum several times a day

■ Defecation occurs as a result of the interaction of several different parts of the nervous system, which cause the pelvic and rectal muscles to contract and the anal sphincter muscles to relax

What are the symptoms?

How do doctors diagnose IBS?

As there is no laboratory or other test that confirms the diagnosis of IBS, doctors have to rely on the symptoms alone. These vary from person to person, but there are three main types.

The predominant symptom may be painful constipation, or the main problem may be a painless, though worrying and inconvenient, diarrhoea. Also, both types of bowel disturbances can occur together accompanied by abdominal pain.

Additional symptoms may include swelling (distension) of the abdomen with wind and unpredictable, erratic bowel actions varying from day to day.

There are some sex differences: straining and passage of hard stools may occur more commonly in women. In contrast, men are more likely to have frequent, loose stools.

As IBS can be diagnosed only from a collection of symptoms, doctors use certain criteria to help them.

Symptoms of IBS

The symptoms vary from person to person.

There are three main types:

1. Painful constipation

2. Diarrhoea

3. Painful constipation and diarrhoea together, accompanied by abdominal pain

Additional symptoms may include:

- Swelling (distension) of the abdomen with wind

- Unpredictable, erratic bowel actions varying from day to day

- Indigestion (dyspepsia)

The Manning criteria

An early attempt by a doctor called Manning to define IBS came up with a list of symptoms associated with the disorder. This identified six main features:

1. Abdominal pain relieved by defecation (bowel action)

2. Looser stools with the onset of abdominal pain

3. More frequent stools with the onset of abdominal pain

4. Abdominal distension

5. Passage of mucus in stools

6. Sensation of incomplete evacuation of the bowel.

The Rome criteria

More recently, an international team of gastro-enterologists listed further symptoms, known as the Rome criteria. These recommend that a diagnosis of IBS be made when someone has had abdominal discomfort or pain for at least 12 weeks in the previous 12 months and the pain or discomfort shows two of the following features:

1. The pain is relieved with defecation.

2. Onset of pain is associated with a change in frequency of passing stools.

3. Onset of pain is associated with a change in form (appearance) of stools.

According to the Rome criteria, the diagnosis of IBS is strengthened by the occurrence of further symptoms. People with constipation as the main symptom may have fewer than three bowel movements a week, with hard or lumpy stools. In contrast, those with diarrhoea as the main symptom may have three or more bowel movements in a day with loose (mushy) or watery stools.

Other symptoms seen in IBS

Other symptoms include:

- straining during bowel movements
- urgency (having to rush to have a bowel movement)
- having a feeling of incomplete bowel movement
- passing mucus or slime with the bowel movement
- having abdominal fullness, bloating or swelling.

Non-gastrointestinal features

A wide range of non-gastrointestinal features may also be associated with IBS (see box on page 18). In addition, about 90 per cent of people with IBS also have dyspepsia (indigestion). Symptoms can vary over the years from being mainly bowel-type to mainly indigestion-type symptoms.

Quality of life

Medically speaking, IBS is not a life-threatening condition. However, if you are a sufferer you will know how much it can restrict your social activities and reduce your quality of life. Chronic food-related pain may mean that you have to avoid going out to eat with friends or family. Fears about the need to open your bowels frequently may seriously limit what you feel able to do.

Restricting activities

Over 40 per cent of people with IBS say that they avoid some activities as a result of their symptoms. Examples are: travelling, socialising, sexual intercourse, domestic and leisure activities, or eating certain foods. Often it is this disruption of normal life rather than individual symptoms as such that determines how you rate the severity of your condition.

Effects on well-being

People with IBS often also experience anxiety and disturbed sleep, with associated lethargy and an inability to get on with their lives. These symptoms can easily start to dominate a sufferer's existence.

If your doctor is unable to diagnose the cause of your symptoms easily, you are likely to be worried.

Non-gastrointestinal features of IBS

A wide range of other problems may occur along with the more typical ones of IBS. Women may have gynaecological problems, there may be a problem passing urine or other symptoms that affect well-being.

Gynaecological symptoms

- Painful periods (dysmenorrhoea)
- Pain after sexual intercourse (dyspareunia)
- Premenstrual tension

Urinary symptoms

- Frequency – needing to urinate often
- Urgency – not being able to wait to urinate
- Passing urine at night (nocturia)
- Incomplete emptying of bladder

Other symptoms

- Back pain
- Headaches
- Bad breath
- Unpleasant taste in the mouth
- Poor quality of sleep
- Constant tiredness
- Depression
- Anxiety
- Fibromyalgia

You may have to keep going back to your GP and/or the hospital outpatient clinic for unpleasant tests.

Sometimes, especially if you are a woman, you may end up having unnecessary surgery in an attempt to improve persistent symptoms. This may be removal of your gallbladder or uterus. However, surgery can make your existing disorder worse. It may also create its own specific postoperative complications, such as pain in the operation scar and adhesions (internal scarring causing cramping pains).

KEY POINTS

- Your doctor will diagnose IBS if you meet the Manning or the Rome criteria

- A wide range of non-gastrointestinal features is associated with IBS, for example, gynaecological, urinary, musculoskeletal and psychological symptoms

Understanding pain

What causes pain?

Apart from those people whose main symptom is repeated painless diarrhoea, most people with IBS complain of pain. In spite of this their tests show that there is no structural abnormality of the intestines. So what causes the pain?

Pain is often a sign that you are doing something that may damage your body – for example, picking up a hot saucepan handle – or it may remind you that you already have damage from a burn or a bruise and that your body needs time to heal. Throughout the body, there are sensitive nerves which, when stimulated or irritated, send messages to the brain that are perceived as pain. Pain is primarily a protective mechanism, alerting you that something is wrong. It is often this that makes you consult a GP – and once the cause is dealt with it has served its purpose.

Pain is described as acute when it has come on recently (and often suddenly) and chronic if you have had it for a considerable length of time.

Types of abdominal pain

Doctors often find it difficult to distinguish between pain caused by a structural abnormality or disease (organic pain) and pain that does not appear to result from any identifiable structural changes or disease processes (functional pain).

Functional pain

The term 'functional pain' comes from the idea that the pain is the result of changes in the function of part of the body. Functional pain can be just as severe and disabling as organic pain – for example, women may describe their attacks of functional pain related to IBS as worse than that of childbirth.

Most people with IBS experience functional abdominal pain caused by disturbed bowel action. The term 'functional abdominal pain' covers pain originating from any site within the abdominal cavity, including the gastrointestinal tract. Women seem to experience it more than men, particularly around the time of the menopause, when hormonal changes influence muscle activity in the intestines.

Is the pain organic or functional?

Even an experienced doctor may sometimes find it difficult to tell whether your pain is organic or functional. Nevertheless, it is important that the distinction is made, to avoid any possibility of an organic disease (such as a bowel tumour) being wrongly diagnosed as a functional disorder (for example, as IBS).

The problem for the doctor is to distinguish the two types of pain without subjecting you to a series of tests that may be intensive, often uncomfortable, occasionally dangerous and usually expensive. Such tests are not needed for someone with non-organic, functional pain.

On the other hand, doctors have to take care not to dismiss too quickly someone who may have organic pain. Throughout the rest of the book, I explain how doctors use guidelines to help them choose the right approach.

What triggers abdominal pain?

Abdominal organs are usually insensitive to many stimuli that would be very painful if applied to your skin. Cutting, tearing or crushing of the gut, for example, does not result in pain.

However, the nerve endings of pain fibres in the muscular walls of the gut are sensitive to stretching or tension. This means that excessive distension or tight contractions (spasm) in the gut wall will trigger pain.

Visceral and referred pain

There are two types of abdominal pain that can occur

Types of pain in IBS

Pain is a signal that something is wrong. There are many different terms to describe it. Those most often used in IBS are described below.

- Acute: short lasting
- Chronic: long term
- Functional: caused by abnormal functioning
- Organic: the reult of disease
- Visceral: felt in the abdomen
- Referred: felt somewhere other than the source

in IBS. One is visceral pain (pain from the internal organs of the abdomen and intestines). The other is referred pain, which is felt in a different part of the body to the part that triggers the pain.

Visceral pain

Visceral pain is felt in the abdomen as a result of some stimulus within the gut itself. The pain is usually dull and focused mostly somewhere along a line down the middle of the abdomen (the midline). It may be higher up or lower down, depending on where the nerve supply to the affected organ originates.

When volunteers took part in experiments in which a balloon was used to distend different parts of the gut, the pain was felt in the midline of the abdomen. In addition:

- Pain arising from distension of the oesophagus was perceived behind the breastbone.

- Pain from stimulation of the duodenum (the first part of the small intestine) was felt in the solar plexus (between the lower ribs in the midline).

- Pain from the lower part of the small intestine (jejunum and ileum) was felt around the navel.

- Pain resulting from distension of the colon was felt in the midline of the lower abdomen.

In these studies there was no mention of pain caused by the balloons being felt anywhere outside the abdominal area. These findings correspond closely with the pattern of abdominal pain experienced by people with organic diseases. The distribution of pain felt by people with functional abdominal pain, however, is much less clear cut and often unusual compared with

Where you feel organic abdominal pain

The source of the pain may be to one side of your body. However, it is usually felt in the midline. If felt in the solar plexus it may be from the stomach, pancreas, gallbladder or duodenum. If felt around the navel, it may be from the small intestine or ascending colon. If felt in the lower abdomen, it may be from the colon, ovary, uterus, kidney or bladder.

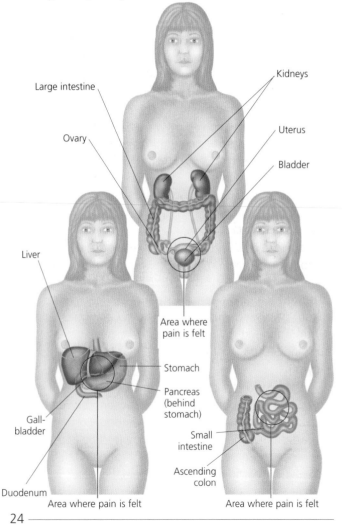

Kidneys

Large intestine

Ovary

Uterus

Bladder

Liver

Area where
pain is felt

Stomach

Pancreas
(behind
stomach)

Gall-
bladder

Small
intestine

Ascending
colon

Duodenum

Area where pain is felt

Area where pain is felt

the abdominal pain experienced by people with organic diseases (see page 24).

Referred pain

Referred pain is felt in an area that may be some distance away from the area where it is actually being caused. This happens when the brain interprets signals from one part of the body as coming from another area. It does this when another area is supplied by the same nerve pathways as the organ involved. One example is pain caused by gallstones which is often felt between the shoulder blades.

Referred pain may be felt in skin or deeper tissues, but is usually confined to one particular area. Sometimes, the skin covering the painful region becomes unusually sensitive, and underlying muscles may feel tender or painful.

Pain threshold

The pain threshold is the level of tolerance at which someone perceives discomfort as pain. Some people have a low pain threshold and can tolerate less discomfort than others with a high pain threshold.

Your pain threshold is a subjective factor which can vary from time to time. It depends on circumstances, your mood, the real or assumed cause of the pain, and many other influences.

Common myths about chronic pain

If they can't find a reason for my pain it must all be in my head!

Sometimes the cause of pain isn't clear – but the pain is still very real. Fortunately there is a lot that you can do to help yourself live with pain, even if you do not know the cause.

Maybe if I ignore the pain it will just go away?

No! Some effort and learning are necessary to manage pain effectively.

Perhaps I am suffering with this pain because I am a bad person?

Long-lasting (chronic) pain isn't a punishment for your past. But the things that you do and the way that you behave have an important effect on your self-esteem and the way that you feel.

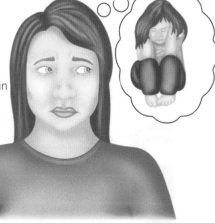

Common myths about chronic pain (contd)

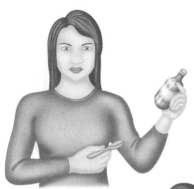

There are drugs that can cure pain.

Drugs can be effective in relieving pain. No drugs cure pain permanently.

Some people pretend to have pain as an excuse not to work or to get sympathy.

A few people may fake pain, but most sufferers of chronic pain only want relief.

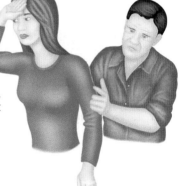

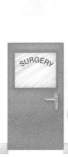
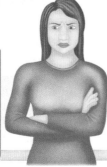

My doctors don't care, otherwise they would do something about my pain.

Your doctors will do everything that they can to assist you and relieve your pain. If they aren't completely successful, it isn't because they don't care.

27

What can influence the severity of IBS symptoms?

Various factors can play a part in determining the severity of the symptoms of IBS; some relate to the illness itself, others to individual circumstances.

These include:

Your personality
Psychological factors
Worry about your illness
Impaired ability to express emotions
Stress levels
Depression, anxiety or panic attacks

The form your condition takes
Chronic (long lasting) or intermittent
Unusual symptoms
Symptoms poorly controlled

Your circumstances
Poor social circumstances
Attitudes of relatives and friends
Sexual abuse as a child
Work and personal satisfaction
Economic gains from having an illness
Medical investigation and treatment

KEY POINTS

- Pain is a subjective sensation felt when nervous impulses from a tissue or organ are transmitted to the brain

- Pain may be acute (sudden onset) or chronic (long term)

- Pain may be organic or functional; most people with IBS get functional abdominal pain

- Pain may be felt in the abdomen (visceral) or somewhere unrelated (referred)

- Your pain threshold is influenced by your circumstances, mood, the real or assumed cause of your pain, and many other factors

Causes of IBS

What triggers IBS?

The gastrointestinal tract is designed to digest food and propel the unabsorbed waste products to the end of the intestines for excretion. It does this by coordinated contraction and relaxation of the muscles in the bowel wall.

Although we do not completely understand the cause of IBS, one factor is disordered contractions of these bowel muscles. It is because the abnormalities involve bowel function, rather than any structural damage or abnormality, that IBS is often described as a functional disorder.

Why should some people develop IBS, whereas others do not? We do not know all the answers to that question, although some factors have been identified that are associated with an increased likelihood that an individual will have IBS. The main factors are:

- psychological factors
- abnormal activity of the bowel muscles and nerves

- increased sensitivity of the gut
- gastrointestinal infections
- diet, food intolerance and food allergy.

Who consults a doctor?

By no means everyone with symptoms consistent with
IBS consults their doctor; the proportion ranges from
10 to 50 per cent, and is influenced by age and sex.
Some people find that their symptoms are troublesome
whereas others pay them little attention.

Studies that have looked at the reasons why people
go to the doctor have found both physical and
psychological differences between those who complain
of their symptoms and those who do not. As you
might expect, people with more symptoms and more
severe pain are more likely to complain, as are those
with psychological symptoms such as anxiety and
depression.

Psychological factors

People with IBS symptoms who do not consult a
doctor are no more or less likely to experience
psychological symptoms than those who don't have
the condition. Around 8 to 15 per cent of people who
consult their GP about their IBS symptoms have
psychological symptoms, which is only a slightly higher
percentage than among people without IBS.

However, psychological symptoms are much more
common in people who are referred to a
gastroenterology clinic. They also seem to be more
common in people with IBS attending hospital than in
a comparable group of people with an inflammatory
bowel disease (IBD) such as Crohn's disease or
ulcerative colitis.

How the bowel muscles work

When the muscles in the bowel wall contract, they move the contents along. When short sections contract and then relax, the contents move back and forth. If the contractions follow each other in a wave along the length of the bowel, the contents are moved towards the rectum. The difference is not in the strength of the contraction but in whether it keeps moving in the same direction, towards the rectum.

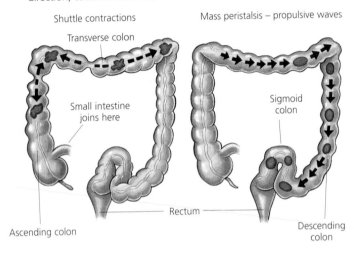

Shuttle contractions

Mass peristalsis – propulsive waves

Transverse colon

Small intestine joins here

Sigmoid colon

Rectum

Ascending colon

Descending colon

Several studies have also found a link between the onset of IBS symptoms and a preceding stressful event such as employment difficulties, bereavement, marital stress or an operation. Some studies have also found links between the development of IBS symptoms and social problems relating to work, finances, housing or personal relationships.

These findings suggest that an individual's mood and emotions influence the way that they respond to their symptoms (for example, whether they consult a doctor), as well as having a direct effect on their intestines. Stress has also been shown to play an important role in causing intestinal pain.

Nevertheless, despite these findings, many people with IBS do not have any obvious psychological or personality problems.

Depression and IBS

Around 10 to 15 per cent of people with IBS who are referred to gastroenterology clinics are found to have a serious depressive illness and a minority of these may even be suicidal. This is why your doctor will want to ask you about symptoms that might suggest that you are depressed – such as sleep disturbance, low mood and changes in energy. However, the detection of depression is sometimes more difficult and, if your doctor is concerned, you may be referred for a full psychiatric assessment. If depression is present, recognised and treated, pain will often disappear, even if severe.

Influence of mood on the gut

When you're depressed, the passage of waste matter throughout your whole gut is likely to be delayed. In contrast, anxiety is associated with accelerated passage of the digestive contents through the small bowel.

Most people have, at some time or other, experienced cramps and diarrhoea caused by major anxiety. Acute stress also accelerates the passage of bowel contents through the small intestine and speeds up the working of the whole colon, so you have to open your bowels more often, whether or not you have IBS.

Research has shown that pain may be made less distressing by techniques such as relaxation and hypnosis. On the other hand, hyperventilation (rapid breathing that occurs during anxiety and panic attacks) has been shown to lower your pain threshold, so that any pain becomes more troublesome.

Abnormal activity of the bowel muscles and nerves

The workings of your bowels are controlled by several different parts of your nervous system. Changes in the activity of the nerves that supply the gut have been found in people with IBS. Abnormal action in one part of the nerve supply (the vagus nerve) is linked to constipation, whereas in another part (known as the sympathetic nervous system) it is linked to diarrhoea. Psychological factors can affect these nerves and so can alter the speed at which intestinal contents pass through the bowels.

People who are constipated, including those with IBS for whom this symptom predominates, seem to have weaker and fewer contraction waves in their colonic muscle. However, there is another group who have increased contractions in the last part of the colon.

Studies have generally shown fast passage of bowel contents in diarrhoea-predominant IBS and slow transit time in constipation-predominant IBS. Some people with IBS may also experience abnormalities in small bowel contraction.

Abnormal bursts of nerve and muscle activity in the colon have been linked to episodes of pain in some individuals. In people with functional abdominal pain, the normal stresses of everyday life may provoke unusual muscle and nerve reactions in the stomach and small intestine.

Despite these observations, the relationship between nerve–muscle disturbances in the gut and abdominal pain is not clear cut. Nor is it known whether such disturbances are the result of an abnormality in gut muscle or nerve activity or whether they are triggered by some other abnormal stimulus.

Gastrocolonic response

When we eat, our food stimulates an increase in colonic nerve and muscle activity, which is called the gastrocolonic response or reflex. This effect is one of the main reasons why a baby tends to fill his or her nappy after a meal. This reflex is mainly stimulated by the fat content of food which explains why people with IBS can experience pain after eating, especially after fatty meals.

The gastrocolonic response

When we eat, our food stimulates an increase in colonic nerve and muscle activity, called the gastrocolonic response. This effect is one of the main reasons why babies tend to fill their nappies after a meal.

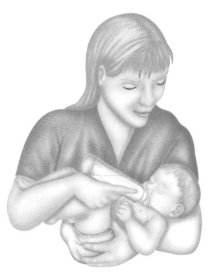

Increased sensitivity of the gut

Studies have been made using balloons inflated in parts of patients' guts to study the pain responses of people with IBS. These have shown that such people are more sensitive than others to distension (or stretching).

In people with IBS, this abnormal sensitivity has been found in all parts of the gastrointestinal tract (oesophagus and small and large intestines). It was also found that trigger areas for the production of pain may occur in the upper, mid and lower gut in the same person.

Pain may be experienced anywhere in the abdomen. It may also be referred to various parts of the body away from the abdomen, such as the back, thigh and arms.

People with functional abdominal pain resulting from IBS have increased sensitivity to the pain caused by the gut being distended with gas, yet their reactions to pain stimuli in other parts of the body are unaffected. They may describe gut stimuli as unpleasant or painful at lower levels of intensity than people who do not have IBS. However, their pain thresholds when subjected to extreme cold or electrical stimulation of the skin may be normal or even increased.

No one knows why this should be the case, but the explanation probably originates in the brain and the way that different types of painful stimuli are perceived.

Gastrointestinal infections

Sometimes, symptoms of IBS can come on after an acute episode of vomiting and diarrhoea. Persistent problems with bowel function (bowel dysfunction) affect around one in four people after food poisoning caused by bacteria such as *Campylobacter*, *Shigella* and *Salmonella* species.

Factors that make persisting symptoms more likely include a more severe acute illness. Examples are:

- diarrhoea lasting more than seven days
- vomiting leading to weight loss
- severe abdominal pain and mucus in the stools.

Other factors are higher anxiety levels and a higher number of stressful events in the six months before the illness.

These types of infection are responsible for long-term symptoms in up to 25 per cent of people with IBS. Such people have a good outlook (prognosis) in that their symptoms often improve or disappear within a year or so.

Diet, food intolerance and food allergy

Eating, especially fatty food, triggers functional abdominal pain in around three of four people with IBS. It is important to distinguish this generalised intolerance to food from intolerance to specific foods, which may produce symptoms in certain individuals.

The role of true (specific) intolerance as a cause of the IBS is debatable. True food intolerance is an adverse reaction in the intestines to a particular food and will occur every time a person eats that particular food. One example of this is excess gas and diarrhoea as a result of lactose intolerance (inability to digest the sugar in milk, see below).

Food allergy, by contrast, brings on immediate symptoms whenever the individual eats the trigger food, such as strawberries or oysters. These allergic symptoms may involve the digestive system (such as vomiting), but they often affect other parts of the body, causing a rash, an attack of asthma or a running nose.

Food intolerance

Studies were made that tested people's response to individual foods by excluding them from the people's diets and then reintroducing them one at a time. These studies found specific food intolerance in between a third and two-thirds of people with IBS. The most common intolerance reported in the UK is to wheat, followed by dairy products (especially cheese, yoghurt and milk), coffee, potato, corn, onions, beef, oats and white wine.

Some people develop typical IBS symptoms such as bloating, cramps and diarrhoea after eating carbohydrates that they are unable to absorb. Examples are lactose (milk sugar) and fructose (fruit sugar). If they are not absorbed, they may ferment in the gut and produce gas. Excluding these from the diet can reduce symptoms and also reduce colonic gas production.

This suggests that changing what you eat can affect the fermentation resulting from the action of bacteria in the colon.

Reduced production of lactase – an enzyme that breaks down lactose – in the lining of the small intestine can develop in adults and is relatively common in the UK. It is estimated to affect 10 per cent of those of northern European descent, rising to 60 per cent in people of Asian origin and 90 per cent of people of Chinese descent.

People taking a substantial amount of lactose (equivalent to more than half a pint of milk per day) can expect to benefit from lactose restriction. On the other hand, those with lower lactose intakes may not, because a low intake does not usually cause symptoms of intolerance.

Elimination diets

An initial study using elimination diets (that is, diets that exclude all but a single type of fruit, a single type of meat, a single vegetable, and so on) improved symptoms in two-thirds of those who completed the study.

More practical elimination diets, which impose less drastic restrictions on what you can eat, have been developed. These exclude only foods that are commonly implicated in food intolerance. These diets have a lower success rate (around 50 per cent) but are easier to follow.

Whether diets for food intolerance are really worthwhile is hard to assess. This is because of the placebo response (in which you feel better just because you are expecting to). Such an effect cannot be ruled out unless foods are given in such a way that neither you nor the researcher knows what you have just eaten when your response is assessed.

Even if you were to be given nothing but blended foods through a tube passing from your nose into your stomach, it is still impossible to assess any particular influences. Examples of such influences are the role played by the important social, psychological and physical aspects of eating. These are likely to be at least as significant as the direct effects of individual foods on the gut. Interestingly, however, a study in which people were fed in this way with suspect food reported that 6 of 25 people with IBS correctly recognised that they had been given one of the foods that seemed to trigger their intolerance.

Specific food intolerance does appear to be the cause of symptoms in a small number of people with IBS. If your doctor suspects that this may be so in your case, you should ideally be referred to a specialist centre for objective, scientifically controlled tests. An enthusiastic, determined approach is required by everyone involved – you, the doctors and dietitians – because these studies need to be conducted for a number of weeks or months.

Food allergy

True food allergy is much less common than food intolerance and is usually not difficult to recognise. This is especially so when eating a particular food (or foods) is associated with a rash, asthma or a running nose.

Such allergies often give a high incidence (70 per cent) of positive results to allergy tests such as skin-prick and blood tests. If you have this type of allergy, you are more likely to see a specialist in immunology rather than a gastroenterologist because your doctor is unlikely to think that you have IBS.

One study tested people with purely intestinal symptoms. It found that only 15 of 88 people who believed that they had a food allergy had this confirmed in a double-masked trial (a trial in which neither they nor the tester knew what food they were eating). Skin-prick tests are more likely to be positive if your symptoms come on immediately after eating the suspect food than if they develop only some hours later.

Women and IBS

Although men and women in general are equally likely to develop IBS, studies have shown that women tend to consult their doctor more often than men. Anxiety, depression and stress are known to occur more often in women, and this may play a part in triggering

Skin-prick test for allergy

A skin-prick test involves the tester placing drops of the suspect allergens on the skin. The skin is then pricked through each drop with a fine needle. An allergic reaction produces a red, itchy weal.

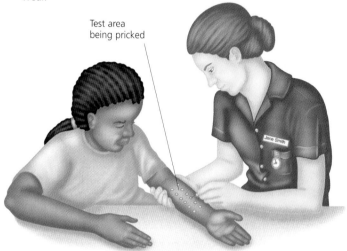

Test area being pricked

symptoms. It is also possible that hormonal differences may contribute to the differences between the sexes. During menstruation, for example, IBS symptoms of abdominal pain, diarrhoea and gas tend to get worse in 50 per cent of women.

Women with IBS are also more likely than men to show increased sensitivity of the gut and three times more likely than men to develop IBS after a gastrointestinal infection.

In 60 per cent of women with IBS, pain may also sometimes be felt deep in the pelvis following intercourse. It can come on several hours after intercourse, particularly when the woman has constipation.

KEY POINTS

■ There are a number of factors, both physiological and psychological, that may make an individual more susceptible to IBS

■ Many people who develop IBS symptoms have had stressful experiences, such as work difficulties, bereavement, marital problems and operations, in the preceding months

■ People who develop IBS after a gut infection tend to have a better prognosis

■ Three-quarters of people with IBS experience abdominal pain after eating, and a small proportion of them are intolerant to specific foods

■ Women are more prone to IBS than men

Getting a diagnosis

Consulting your GP about abdominal pain

Functional abdominal pain is common, but only about half the people affected actually consult their GP and, of these, only about one in five is referred to a hospital consultant in any given year.

If you consult your GP about abdominal pain, he or she will ask a variety of questions. These are to assess your symptoms, psychological state and social circumstances, as well as your past family and personal history. If you are under the age of 45 with typical symptoms of IBS (see page 15) and appear normal on physical examination, you may not need further investigations. Your doctor may suggest further tests to rule out other bowel problems (see pages 45–6) if you have weight loss, rectal bleeding or symptoms responsible for night-time waking, or if your symptoms have come on suddenly over a relatively short period of time.

Otherwise, your doctor will give you a full physical examination. This may include a rectal examination using a small viewing instrument to look inside your

Examination of the rectum with a sigmoidoscope

The patient lies on the side with the knees bent. The instrument is carefully inserted into the rectum. The light source helps the doctor to see any abnormalities in the rectum and lower colon.

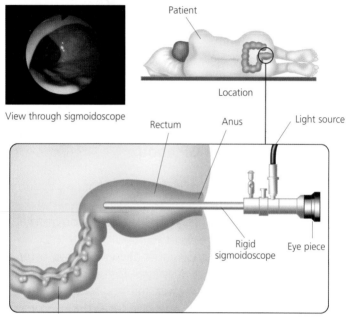

View through sigmoidoscope

Patient

Location

Rectum

Anus

Light source

Rigid sigmoidoscope

Eye piece

Sigmoid colon

rectum and lower colon (sigmoidoscopy). These examinations, together with what you have told the doctor about your symptoms, should be sufficient for a diagnosis to be made. Sometimes, a doctor may slightly expand your rectum with air. This can reassure you of the diagnosis by demonstrating that it is just distension that is triggering your pain.

What happens if IBS is diagnosed?

If you have a typical history of IBS (your symptoms meet the Manning or Rome criteria, with or without negative test results), your doctor will usually confirm the diagnosis of IBS and give you a detailed explanation of the condition. He or she will reassure you that most symptoms disappear on their own or at least become tolerable once you understand what is causing them.

Your doctor may also suggest simple drug treatments or dietary changes that may help (see pages 98–102). You may also be recommended to use psychological therapies such as relaxation (see page 96).

If your symptoms continue, however, you will be reviewed regularly. It is important that a doctor makes the diagnosis of IBS – this is not a diagnosis you should ever make yourself.

When will your GP refer you to hospital?

This is likely to be necessary if you have developed bowel symptoms for the first time in later life, or if your symptoms are not typical of someone with IBS. If you have had IBS for a while and your symptoms become worse, or new features appear, you may also be referred to a specialist, both to rule out other possible bowel conditions and to provide greater reassurance than your GP can offer.

Hospital investigations

Over the last 30 years, a variety of new tests has become available to help identify or exclude organic disease. These include endoscopy (examining the internal organs with a viewing instrument sometimes incorporating a tiny camera) and scanning techniques. These investigations are done in a hospital. A sedative may be given before some types of endoscopy.

One approach to assessing abdominal pain is therefore to perform a series of endoscopic and scanning examinations. Only if all these yield negative results is functional pain or IBS diagnosed.

Disadvantage of hospital investigations

Although extensive investigations may sometimes be necessary in difficult cases, most people don't really need them and they have a number of disadvantages. From your point of view, the process can be very demoralising. It can increase your anxiety that there may be something seriously wrong and undermine your confidence in your doctor as each test comes up with negative results.

It's not unusual for such investigations to detect another condition, such as a hiatus hernia (weakness in the diaphragm muscle), which in fact is not responsible for your symptoms. If doctors decide to treat such a problem, sometimes with an operation, your IBS symptoms may disappear for a short time. However, they will invariably come back, and you will then have to cope with them as well as any consequences of the surgery.

Fortunately, functional pain caused by IBS is much more common than organic pain resulting from inflammatory bowel disease. For this reason, your doctor will usually be able to make a positive diagnosis based on your symptoms and a physical examination alone, without the need for extensive investigations.

Other symptoms

Although the diagnosis of IBS is based on medically agreed criteria (see page 15), many people do have additional symptoms, and you should mention to your GP any that you have. As well as abdominal pain, common associated symptoms include nausea,

Examination of rectum and colon with a colonoscope

The patient lies on the side with the knees bent, and usually has a mild sedative. The colon has previously been emptied, by not eating, flushing out the contents using medication and drinking large quantities of fluid. The flexible tube is inserted slowly along the colon and the small internal camera is connected to a video screen. In this diagram, the tube has reached the ascending colon.

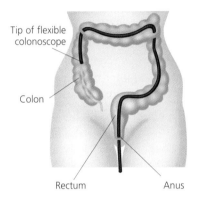

Tip of flexible colonoscope

Colon

Rectum

Anus

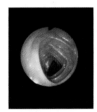

The display on the video screen shows the lining of the colon

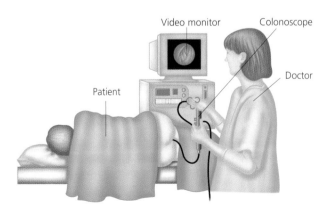

Video monitor

Colonoscope

Doctor

Patient

vomiting, difficulty swallowing (dysphagia) and a feeling of fullness after eating.

You may notice the passage of undigested food in the faeces. This usually consists of vegetable residues such as tomato skins or corn and merely indicates rapid transit through the gastrointestinal tract.

Non-gastrointestinal symptoms that people with IBS may also experience include regularly passing urine at night, needing to do so frequently and urgently, and the feeling that you are unable to empty your bladder completely. Some people also experience back pain, an unpleasant taste in the mouth and a constant feeling of tiredness, and women may find intercourse painful.

If you have lost weight, your doctor may want to arrange some investigations to rule out a serious bowel problem. He or she may also ask questions to assess your mental state because depression may lead to a loss of weight.

Gynaecological disorders

Your doctor will want to rule out other causes of lower abdominal and pelvic pain. For women, there are several gynaecological disorders that may also cause pain in the lower abdomen and the pelvis (the bony funnel that contains the bladder, rectum and internal female reproductive organs). These disorders include:

- Pelvic inflammatory disease – inflammation of the tubes connecting the ovaries to the uterus (the fallopian tubes) and other structures in the pelvis.

- Endometriosis – in which cells from the lining of the womb are found in the pelvis.

- Pain that occurs in the middle of the menstrual cycle caused by swelling followed by rupture of a ripening egg follicle.

- Occasionally, pain in the lower abdomen and disturbed bowel function could be a symptom of cancer of the cervix or the ovaries, and if your doctor thinks that either of these is a possibility, he or she may arrange for you to see a gynaecologist. However, such cancers are very rare compared with IBS.

KEY POINTS

■ Your GP will need as much information as you can give about your pain; it is worth making a note in advance so that you can tell him or her what brings it on, makes it worse or better, where the pain is and whether it spreads to other parts of your body

■ Although some people may need further investigations in a hospital clinic, often your GP will be able to make the diagnosis of IBS using the Manning or Rome criteria

■ When you see your GP, you will be asked questions about your lifestyle and any recent stressful events because psychological factors can play an important part in IBS

■ Most people with IBS will be looked after by their GP without needing to attend a hospital outpatient clinic

Constipation

What is a normal bowel habit?

People vary a lot in how often they open their bowels – usually between three times a day and three times a week in the UK. Interestingly, people living in different parts of the country and people from different ethnic backgrounds may have different bowel habits, possibly because of variations in their diets. A stool should be solid, but moist and easy to pass.

How the bowel works

Contraction and relaxation of the colon and rectum are regulated by three separate parts of the nervous system (sympathetic, parasympathetic and enteric nervous systems). Physical disorders affecting these pathways will influence how often you need to open your bowels. The activity of muscles in the colon is also stimulated by factors such as food and emotion.

When there are sufficient faeces in the rectum to distend it, this causes its smooth muscle to contract in a reflex action and also makes the internal sphincter muscles (which keep the anus closed) relax. The stool is

What does the bowel do?

Food passes from the stomach to the small intestine and then to the large intestine. We absorb nutrients from the digested food and most of the fluids that we have drunk. Some of this fluid is from intestinal secretions. The remaining waste matter (faeces) is pushed to the rectum where we expel it through the anus. The bowel:

- Receives the food and liquids that we eat and drink

- Increases the amount of fluid in the intestines by liquid secretions from its lining

- Propels food contents from the stomach down its length to the back passage (anus)

- Absorbs most of the nutrients from our food and drink into the bloodstream

- Excretes waste material as stools

then expelled when we contract the diaphragm and abdominal muscles, and relax the pelvic floor muscles and external sphincter muscles.

What is constipation?

Constipation is largely a subjective sensation and has no universally accepted definition. A person can be considered to be constipated when fewer than three bowel actions happen in a week, or if there is often a need to strain to pass a stool.

Constipation is hardly ever harmful in that you won't become 'poisoned' or 'dirty' if your bowels don't open. Although constipation is not a disease, it is occasionally a symptom of an underlying disease.

What causes the usual types of constipation?

There are several simple explanations for most constipation. It is often caused by an unsuitable diet, bad bowel habits or not using the muscles effectively:

- Diet: usually a lack of fibre (roughage) in the diet.

- Bad bowel habits: most people have an urge to go to the toilet once or twice a day. This often happens after a meal. If this urge is ignored, the stool dries out and becomes hard. The next bowel movement may then be difficult or painful.

- Uncoordinated straining: some people do not strain effectively and/or fail to relax the muscles around the back passage when they strain.

Your abdomen may feel uncomfortable or bloated and you may have a sense of fullness above your back passage (rectum and anus). Straining can lead to piles (see page 57), which may bulge at the anus or bleed. Women may also find intercourse uncomfortable if the bowel is very full.

What causes constipation?

The most common causes of constipation are simple and easily put right. If your diet does not contain enough fibre, it is more difficult for your bowel to pass food along and keep the faeces soft enough to pass easily.

Modern lifestyles make it difficult to respond immediately to the urge to empty your bowels. Ignoring this urge means that the faeces are stored longer and they can become hard and dry.

Some people do not strain effectively or fail to relax the anal muscle to allow the rectum to empty. Retraining the use of the muscles will help this problem.

What makes constipation worse?

Your bowel function is affected by many factors. These can make any tendency to constipation worse.

You must drink enough fluid each day – about two litres. If you become dehydrated, your faeces will become harder.

Physical exercise massages the bowels and helps the passage along the gut, so inactivity will make any constipation worse.

Your emotions have a strong effect on your bowels. Anxiety can speed the passage along your bowels, but other emotions can slow it down and lead to constipation.

Painful conditions that affect the anus will aggravate any constipation. Piles are the result of straining, which you are more likely to do if you are

What factors can aggravate constipation?

If you have a tendency to constipation, there are many factors that can make it worse:

- Dehydration: low fluid levels in the body
- Inactivity – lack of exercise
- Emotional upsets
- Painful anal conditions such as piles
- Shift work
- Lack of toilet facilities

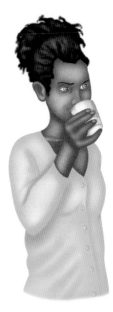

Drink plenty of fluids, at least four pints spread over the day.

constipated. As they are painful it makes it harder to respond to a need to empty the bowels.

Working hours can interfere with a regular bowel habit. You may have to be at work early in the morning and leave home before you have emptied your bowels. Or you may work shifts that interfere with your normal body rhythm.

A lack of suitable toilet facilities can aggravate constipation. Many people need to feel comfortable before they can empty their bowels.

What disorders cause constipation?

A number of organic and functional disorders can affect bowel movement. Any obstruction of the bowel as a result of scarring or inflammation or the growth of a tumour can lead to constipation. The pressure of an enlarged uterus and other changes in pregnancy can affect bowel movement. An underactive thyroid gland often results in constipation. Any alteration in the nerves or muscles that control bowel movement, as happens in IBS, can lead to constipation.

What conditions and disorders may cause constipation?

There may be underlying organic or functional reasons for constipation:

- Obstruction to the bowels by scarring, inflammation or a tumour

- Pregnancy

- Underactive thyroid gland

- Altered function in the nerves or muscles controlling bowel movement, such as in IBS

What medicines cause constipation?

Medications all have some effects other than those for which we take them. One of the side effects is constipation. All side effects from medication should be explained on the patient information leaflet that comes with the medication. Those medications that are known to be likely to cause constipation are listed in the box on page 56.

What is fibre and how does it help?

Fibre is found in the tough fibrous part of fruit and vegetables. In particular it is found in the stalk and on

What medicines can cause constipation?

Some constipation can be a side effect of medication taken for another reason. This is usually explained on the patient information leaflet that comes with the medication:

- Antacids that contain aluminium or calcium taken for indigestion

- Iron tablets (sometimes)

- Some pain-killers such as codeine

- Cough medicines that also contain codeine

- 'Nerve' treatments:
  - some antidepressant drugs
  - certain tranquillisers

- Drugs that influence muscle function, such as some given for abdominal pain, bladder relaxation or Parkinson's disease

the outside of fruits, seeds or grains (bran is the outer covering of wheat grains). It is also in the soft parts of fruit and vegetables that are not digested by the small intestine.

Much of the food that we eat is digested in the stomach and small intestine and is absorbed as nutrients. Fibre is not broken down in this way but passes to the large intestine (colon). Here it:

- acts like blotting paper, keeping water in the stool

- provides material that encourages the multiplication of useful bacteria in the colon.

Haemorrhoids (piles)

Piles (haemorrhoids) are anal blood vessels that have been pushed down and may protrude from the anal canal. Piles are caused by straining to pass a stool.

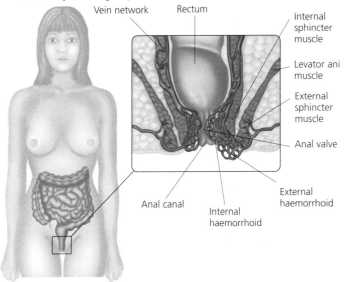

Vein network · Rectum · Internal sphincter muscle · Levator ani muscle · External sphincter muscle · Anal valve · External haemorrhoid · Anal canal · Internal haemorrhoid

Both these effects make the stool larger, softer and easier to pass. Bulky stools stimulate your gut wall, increasing the propulsive waves of contraction (peristalsis) so that they pass through more easily.

Dietary fibre is found only in foods that come from plants – for example, cereals, fruit and vegetables. It is not found in animal foods. So, if you need to increase your fibre intake, gradually start to use the foods listed on pages 58–61. If you already eat some of them, try to do so more often.

You may experience some increase in the amount of gas in the intestines (flatulence) and this may lead to abdominal discomfort at first. This should lessen as your body becomes used to the change in your diet.

Drink plenty of fluids (at least four pints a day) because the fibre will absorb water. It may be helpful to discuss what you eat with a dietitian.

Foods containing a good source of fibre

There is a wide variety of appetising foods that contain fibre. They are all foods that come from plants:

- Wholemeal bread: eat this regularly in preference to white, brown or wheatmeal bread or try other varieties such as granary, Hi-bran, high-fibre white and oatbread. You could also try wholemeal muffins, scones, crumpets, pitta bread and chapatis. Bread is good for you, so eat plenty.

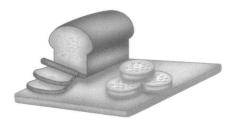

- Wholegrain and high-fibre breakfast cereals: for example, porridge, muesli, Weetabix, Shredded Wheat, Bran Flakes, All Bran. Have some every day.

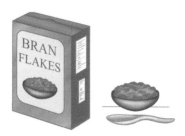

- Wholemeal flour: try using equal quantities of wholemeal flour and white flour in cooking (don't sieve the flour). You will need to add more fluid for pastry and chapatis.

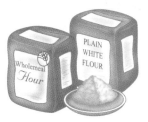

- Biscuits and crackers: instead of biscuits and cream crackers made with white flour, have digestive bran biscuits, flapjacks, oatcakes/oat biscuits, cereal bars, wholewheat crackers and wholegrain crispbreads.

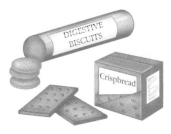

- Brown rice: this takes longer to cook than white rice, but it is more nutritious.

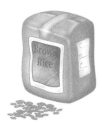

- Wholemeal pasta: for example, spaghetti, macaroni, lasagne.

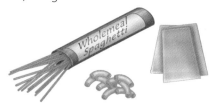

- Pulses: these include dried peas, beans, lentils, dhals and tinned beans. The dried ones need to be soaked and boiled vigorously for at least 10 minutes. They can then be cooked for the remainder of the recommended time. Try using them in soups and to replace some of the meat in stews and casseroles. They can be cooled and used in salads.

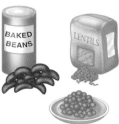

- Vegetables: eat some every day. Wash them well and eat lightly cooked or raw and try crunchy side salads with your main meal and lunchtime snack. Eat plenty of potatoes as they are good for you (especially in their jackets).

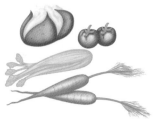

- Fruit: eat fresh (wash well), dried or tinned in natural juices. Eat some every day. Prunes and prune juice are particularly good at relieving constipation. Add dried fruit to cereals and milk puddings, and use in baking.

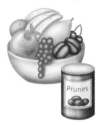

- Nuts and seeds: for example, sunflower seeds. Eat as a snack or use in salads or cooking. Do not give whole nuts to children under five as there is a risk of the child choking or going on to develop a nut allergy.

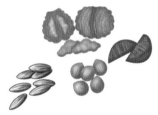

Should I use natural bran?

Natural bran is the outer layer of the wheat grain, not a breakfast cereal. It adds fibre to the diet, but you should use it only if your doctor or a dietitian advises you to do so. It may be useful if your bowels are not regular, even though you eat plenty of the high-fibre foods listed, but should be used only in small amounts.

Start by adding one teaspoon to food or drink at three meals each day. Gradually increase the amount over the next few days if needed. One tablespoon of bran three times daily is usually enough to treat constipation.

Bran can be added to:

- breakfast cereals
- soups, stews, casseroles
- meat and potato pies
- stewed fruit puddings
- drinks (milk or fruit juices).

It may cause some flatulence when you first start to use it.

Dietary fibre, bran and bulk-forming laxatives

Some people with IBS or functional abdominal pain benefit when their doctors prescribe a high-fibre diet, bran or laxatives that add bulk to the stools (bulk-forming laxatives). Others, however, notice no change or even a deterioration in their symptoms.

Bran

There are few studies in which the effect of bran on the symptoms of IBS have been carefully evaluated over long periods. In one such study, bran was found to improve constipation significantly, but it exacerbated diarrhoea, pain and urgency.

Bulk-forming laxatives

Treatment intended to add bulk to the stools is likely to be effective for people who frequently pass small, hard stools or who pass only a painful, irregular stool every few days. A high-fibre diet alone is often ineffective and a bulking agent (a fibre source that swells in the bowels to provide bulk, such as ispaghula husk) is usually required.

Symptoms of gas and pain are sometimes aggravated by an increase in dietary fibre, and therefore it isn't advisable for everyone. If your normal diet is low in fibre, try increasing your intake and adjust the amount according to the way your system responds. On the other hand, especially if your intake is very high and you are experiencing pain and distension, you may need to reduce your intake of fibre.

Combination laxatives

The bulking agent, ispaghula husk, has been shown to be particularly effective in combination with muscle-relaxing (anti-spasmodic) drugs such as hyoscine butylbromide (Buscopan) and mebeverine hydrochloride (Colofac) (see page 99).

What if some foods don't suit me?

Some people with IBS find that pulses, nuts, dried fruits and some vegetables cause a lot of wind or discomfort. If you find that these foods upset you, it may be better to avoid them.

Is it important to eat a breakfast?

Yes. Eating breakfast helps your bowels to start working during the morning.

The best type of breakfast is a wholegrain or high-fibre cereal with some wholemeal toast. If you prefer a cooked breakfast, then perhaps include plenty of wholemeal bread and some baked beans.

Healthy eating can prevent weight increase

If you have to change what you eat to avoid constipation you may be worried about putting on weight. The foods that you will be recommended are not fattening in themselves. You just have to combine them in a healthy and balanced way.

General

- Use a low-fat spread
- Use a low-fat milk
- Take more exercise

Some meal ideas

Breakfast

- Grapefruit or prunes
- Porridge
- Unsweetened muesli
- Weetabix with sliced banana
- Bran flakes
- Wholemeal or granary toast

Snack meals

- Lentil soup and wholemeal roll
- Baked beans on toast or muffin

Healthy eating can prevent weight increase (contd)

- Sandwiches made with wholemeal or high-fibre bread
- Jacket potato with baked beans or sweetcorn filling and a side salad
- Wholemeal pitta bread and humous with salad
- Vegetable and bean soup with a granary roll
- Fresh fruit
- Bran crispbreads, cheese and tomato

Main meals

- Chicken, jacket potato and sweetcorn
- Wholemeal spaghetti bolognese and side salad
- Vegetable curry and brown rice
- Chilli con carne (with red kidney beans) with brown rice and side salad
- Tuna and chick pea salad with granary bread
- Lentil and vegetable casserole with jacket potato
- Grilled fish, jacket potato and peas and sweetcorn
- Vegetables and beans in tomato sauce with wholemeal pasta shapes
- Wholemeal pizza (try adding more vegetables or beans to the topping).

What should you weigh?

• The body mass index (BMI) is a useful measure of healthy weight
• Find out your height in metres and weight in kilograms
• Calculate your BMI like this:

$$BMI = \frac{\text{Your weight (kg)}}{[\text{Your height (metres)} \times \text{Your height (metres)}]}$$

$$\text{e.g. } 24.8 = \frac{70}{[1.68 \times 1.68]}$$

• You are recommended to try to maintain a BMI in the range 20–25
• The chart below is an easier way of estimating your BMI. Read off your height and your weight. The point where the lines cross in the chart indicates your BMI

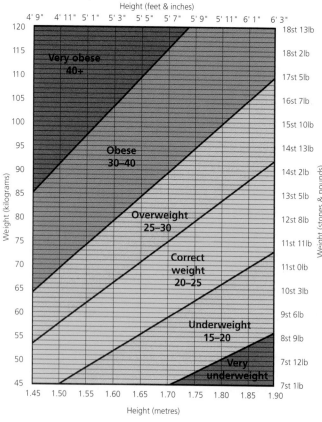

Will I put weight on if I eat more bread, potatoes and cereals?

Not if you cut down your intake of fat, fatty foods, sugar and sweet foods. Bread, potatoes, rice, pasta and cereals are not fattening in themselves, but they are if you serve them with fatty sauces

If you are worried about your weight, try the suggestions in the box on pages 64–5.

For more suggestions, look in your local library or bookshop for books on high-fibre, vegetarian and wholefood cookery.

What if my bowels are not regular?

- Always try to go to the toilet as soon as you feel the urge
- Try to do this as a routine, for example, as soon as you get up, or after breakfast
- Drink at least four pints of fluid daily
- Eat more natural fibre
- Be as active as possible, even if you have a disability
- Avoid laxatives
- Have your meals at the same time every day
- Ensure that you have access to good toilet facilities at home and work
- Take regular exercise.

When should you see your doctor?

If constipation is not responding to these simple self-help measures and is causing you trouble, you should make an appointment to see your doctor. Any changes in bowel habit, either sudden or gradual, should also be reported to the doctor.

You should consult him or her urgently if there is rectal bleeding or new symptoms such as abdominal pain or distension. You should also see your doctor urgently if you suddenly become constipated for no apparent reason.

You will probably not need any tests, although your doctor may want to take a blood sample. This is to make sure that you are not anaemic and that your thyroid gland is working properly. If the constipation is very bad, your doctor may wish to check whether your colon is normal by arranging one of the following at your local hospital:

- A barium enema X-ray: this involves the insertion into the rectum of a harmless material which shows up on an X-ray, allowing the doctor to see any abnormalities.

- A sigmoidoscopy or colonoscopy (inserting a flexible viewing instrument so the doctor can see the interior of the colon) – see pages 44–7.

- Tests to check the function of the muscles around the back passage.

Are laxatives useful?

Constipation is usually improved by a change in your diet, and drugs are therefore not needed. Occasional use of a suitable laxative is harmless, but regular use may make you dependent on it.

Stimulant laxatives, such as senna and cascara, cause changes in the colon if used regularly for many years, but can be useful occasionally for a short time. Laxatives cause gripe-like abdominal pains if used in large doses.

A few people will need to take laxatives regularly, but this should be done only on a doctor's advice.

The most natural and effective types are bulk laxatives. Concentrated fibre preparations are helpful for those who find it hard to change their diet.

The choice of laxatives includes the following:

- Bulk laxatives: bran, ispaghula husk, methylcellulose, sterculia. Always take them with plenty of water. They make stools larger, softer and easier to pass.

- Stimulant laxatives: bisacodyl or senna which stimulates contraction of the bowel.

- Osmotic laxatives: mineral salts (magnesium sulphate/Epsom salts, magnesium citrate, magnesium hydroxide, Movicol, Picolax). These retain water in the bowel, softening the stools and making them easier to pass.

- Lactulose, lactitol or sorbitol sugars which humans cannot digest. They stay in the bowel and combine the properties of bulk and osmotic laxatives.

- Suppositories inserted into the rectum which soften the stool and stimulate bowel action.

- Enemas: a few people, especially those with severe nerve damage in the spine, have to use enemas in which a liquid solution is flushed into the lower bowel to wash it out.

With any laxative, it is important to keep up a good fluid intake – at least four pints of fluid every day and more if possible.

Other treatments

Special tests may show that you have a problem coordinating straining to move the stools while relaxing the exit from the bowel (the anal sphincter). If you have this disorder, you may be helped by training in how to contract your abdominal muscles and relax those around your back passage effectively.

This training can be supplemented by a device that enables you to tell whether your muscle is relaxed (biofeedback – see page 96), but most people don't need this. Training the muscles is, at present, limited to a few centres, but is likely to become more generally available.

If constipation is associated with emotional problems, counselling or similar treatment may help.

A small number of people require surgical treatment, but this is needed only by those with a definite abnormality of the large intestine.

KEY POINTS

■ Changing your diet and developing good bowel habits, together with increased exercise, will be enough for most people to relieve their constipation and control any tendency to gain weight

■ Bulk-forming or osmotic laxatives are preferable to stimulant laxatives, which should be taken regularly only under medical supervision

■ If you are constipated, this does NOT mean that bodily wastes are being absorbed and damaging your health

■ If you are over 40 and for no obvious reason have sudden or gradual changes in bowel habit, you should see your GP (especially if you have rectal bleeding or new abdominal symptoms such as distension)

Diarrhoea

What is diarrhoea?

Diarrhoea means that there are frequent, loose or liquid stools, sometimes accompanied by griping abdominal pain (colic) which lessens after a stool is passed:

- Acute diarrhoea comes on suddenly and lasts a short time.

- Chronic diarrhoea affects someone over a long period of time.

Some people pass frequent, small, solid stools with a sense of urgency. This is not true diarrhoea and occurs when the rectum is irritable as in IBS or inflamed as in colitis.

What causes diarrhoea?

You develop acute diarrhoea when too much fluid is passed (secreted) from the bloodstream into the bowel, for example, in food poisoning or other types of bowel infections. Some laxatives work by provoking a similar response (osmotic laxatives).

Diarrhoea may also be the result of your bowel contents moving through too quickly so that less fluid is passed back into your bloodstream. This is one way in which anxiety produces diarrhoea.

Drinking more liquid than your bowel can cope with can also cause loose motions. Although this seldom happens, it is one way in which drinking too much beer can cause diarrhoea. However, excessive amounts of alcohol can also have the same effect by irritating the bowel. Sometimes treatment with an antibiotic can result in acute diarrhoea.

When diarrhoea goes on for a long time, the most likely cause is IBS. The bowel produces stools that are looser or more frequent than normal, but the bowel is not diseased. You should make an appointment to see your GP if acute diarrhoea does not settle after a few days.

See your doctor promptly if you have severe diarrhoea with dehydration (dry mouth, loose skin, sunken eyes) or if you are over the age of 60. You should ask for an early appointment with your doctor if liquid stools contain blood and/or if you are losing weight.

What will your doctor do?

After asking appropriate questions, and doing a general examination, your doctor will usually examine your rectum (back passage) with a lubricated, gloved finger. Your doctor may:

- pass a viewing instrument (such as a proctoscope or a rigid sigmoidoscope) into your back passage to examine the lining of the bowel (see page 44)

- arrange a laboratory examination of stool samples to see if there is infection

Examination of a stool sample

If your doctor asks for a stool sample to send to the laboratory you will be given a sample pot. At the laboratory the sample will be examined under a microscope to look for any organisms that may cause infection.

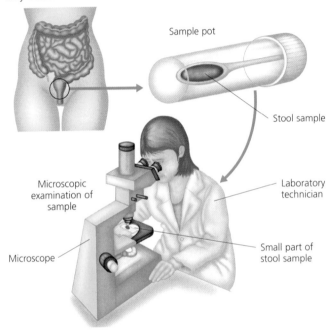

Sample pot

Stool sample

Laboratory technician

Microscopic examination of sample

Microscope

Small part of stool sample

- arrange blood tests

- arrange a barium X-ray examination of your bowel (barium enema)

- arrange an examination of the interior of your colon using a flexible sigmoidoscope or colonoscope and taking samples of the lining for examination if abnormalities are seen (see page 47).

Taking a blood sample

A blood sample is usually taken by a nurse at your GP's surgery. A tourniquet around your upper arm makes the vein stand out. The nurse inserts a small needle into the vein and draws a small sample of blood up into the syringe.

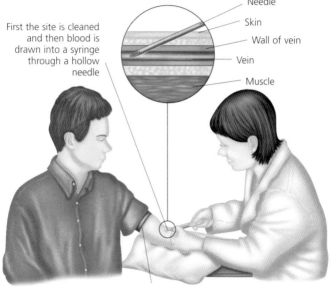

First the site is cleaned and then blood is drawn into a syringe through a hollow needle

Needle

Skin

Wall of vein

Vein

Muscle

A tourniquet may be applied to make the vein more prominent

Drug treatment

Anti-diarrhoeal drugs are helpful if you are passing stools very frequently. However, they may make abdominal discomfort worse and also your constipation worse if you have a tendency to alternate this with bouts of diarrhoea. If taken at night, they may diminish the early morning stool frequency which characterises the 'painless diarrhoea' form of IBS described earlier.

The three common anti-diarrhoeal drugs – codeine phosphate, diphenoxylate (Lomotil) and loperamide

Barium X-ray examination

Your doctor may arrange a barium X-ray examination of your bowel. Barium is a thick liquid that does not allow X-rays to pass through it, so it shows up well on X-ray pictures. It is given as an enema after a laxative has been taken to empty the bowel. X-ray pictures are then taken of the colon.

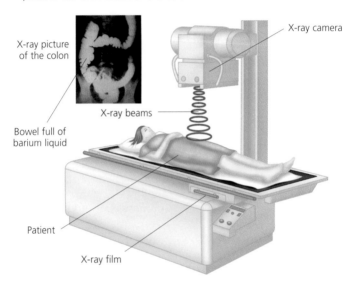

X-ray picture of the colon

X-ray camera

X-ray beams

Bowel full of barium liquid

Patient

X-ray film

(Imodium) – are equally effective in most cases. You may find that one of them suits you better than the others or that one causes fewer side effects.

What is faecal incontinence?

Most of us take it for granted that we can control our bowels. We barely have to think about controlling the release of wind (gas), or of liquid or solid (stools or faeces) from the bowel. We do not have 'accidents' nor are we 'caught short', unless perhaps during a sudden severe bout of diarrhoea.

Sometimes, however, control is lost because the bowel or the muscular ring (sphincter) around the exit from the back passage (anus) does not function properly. Bowel contents escape and this can be extremely embarrassing.

Faecal (or anal) incontinence, also known as soiling, is the loss of stool, liquid or gas from the bowel at an undesirable time. It can occur at any age and may affect up to one in 20 people. It is certainly more common than was thought some years ago. Simple tests can usually show where the problem is, and treatment is often effective.

How do we normally control the bowel?

Normally the bowel and ring of muscle around the back passage (anal sphincter) work together to ensure that bowel contents are not passed until we are ready. The bowel contents move along the bowel gradually.

The sphincter has two main muscles that keep the anus closed. There is an inner ring (internal anal sphincter), which keeps the anus closed at rest, and an outer ring (external anal sphincter), which provides extra protection when we exert ourselves or when we cough or sneeze. These muscles, the nerves supplying them and the sensation felt within the bowel and sphincter all contribute to the sphincter remaining tightly closed. This balance enables us to stay in control (or 'continent').

What causes incontinence?

Faecal incontinence occurs most commonly because the anal sphincter is not functioning properly. Damage to the sphincter muscles or to the nerves controlling these muscles, excessively strong bowel contractions or alterations to bowel sensation can all lead to this disturbance of function.

Men and women of any age may be incontinent for various reasons:

- Children and teenagers – if they are born with an abnormal sphincter or if they have persistent constipation which can affect the sphincter through constant straining.

- Women, after childbirth – usually caused by a tear (hidden or obvious) in the sphincter muscles.

Controlling bowel opening

Faeces are stored in the rectum with its muscular walls relaxed. The anal sphincter is contracted. When we are ready to empty our bowels, we contract the rectal muscles at the same time as relaxing the anal sphincter.

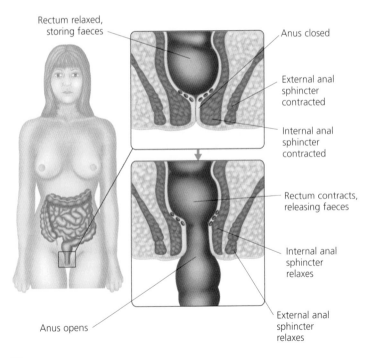

Rectum relaxed, storing faeces

Anus closed

External anal sphincter contracted

Internal anal sphincter contracted

Rectum contracts, releasing faeces

Internal anal sphincter relaxes

Anus opens

External anal sphincter relaxes

- People of any age who experience an injury or infection of the sphincter – they may be affected immediately or later in life.

- People who have inflammatory bowel disease or IBS – because the bowel is very sensitive and squeezes strongly.

- Elderly people – because of constipation and overflow from the bowel as a result of failing mental capacity, or of sphincter damage sustained when they were younger.

- People with disorders such as multiple sclerosis, stroke and epilepsy – which result in damage to the nerves supplying the sphincter.

What tests may be needed?

Tests of sphincter function are relatively simple. They do not require preparation, and are quick to perform and usually pain free.

The strength of the muscles, sensation and nerve function, for example, can all be tested using simple pressure-measuring devices.

An ultrasound scan can provide a clear picture of both the sphincter muscle rings, showing whether one or both are damaged. This test is not uncomfortable, takes only five minutes and involves no radiation.

These tests are performed by doctors with a special interest in continence. If you need them you will be referred by your GP.

What is the treatment?

Anti-diarrhoeal drugs (see page 75) may be helpful when:

- the bowel is squeezing too strongly (an urgent need to get to the toilet quickly)

- the stool is very loose

- the sphincter muscles are weak.

  These drugs can help in several ways:

- decrease movement in the bowel

- make the stool more formed

- make the sphincter muscle tighter.

When the sphincter has been injured, creating a gap in the sphincter muscles, an operation performed through the skin around the anus can often cure the problem. When there is nerve damage to sphincter muscles, a different operation to tighten the sphincter will sometimes help.

Techniques such as biofeedback (see page 96) are now available to retrain the bowel to be more sensitive to the presence of stool, so that the sphincter contracts when necessary.

It is a good idea to plan shopping, outings and so on at times when you feel safest. You can take a 'Can't Wait' card with you (available to members of the IBS Network, see page 110).

KEY POINTS

■ Diarrhoea means frequent, loose or liquid stools; acute diarrhoea usually settles by itself, whereas chronic diarrhoea often requires further investigation, with rectal, barium or endoscope examination of the large bowel

■ IBS is the most common cause of chronic diarrhoea

■ Anti-diarrhoeal drugs, such as codeine, diphenoxylate (Lomotil) and loperamide (Imodium), are usually effective

■ Faecal incontinence is quite common, especially in elderly people and in women who have had difficult and prolonged childbirth; simple tests can often identify these problems and various kinds of treatment are available

Related symptoms

Bad breath

Although an unpleasant smell on the breath (halitosis) may have a variety of organic causes, such as diseases in the mouth and nasal or respiratory tracts, often no such cause can be found. Advice on good oral hygiene may solve the problem for some people, although halitosis can be difficult to treat successfully.

Constipation cannot give you bad breath as some people believe. Psychological or emotional problems may lead some people to believe that they have bad breath when they haven't, and they will need reassurance and possibly treatment for their emotional difficulties.

Unpleasant taste and salivary flow problems

Many of the conditions that cause halitosis may also give you an unpleasant taste in your mouth. A dry mouth, which may be caused by disorders of the salivary glands, drugs or diseases resulting in dehydration, may also be associated with an unpleasant taste. Again, however, symptoms such as this may be the result of anxiety or stress, which make you more likely to breathe through your mouth rather than your nose. If there is no underlying physical cause, you will need the same approach as people with concerns about bad breath.

Some people have the opposite problem and produce too much saliva. This may be caused by dentures or a number of diseases, but it may also be a symptom of a psychological rather than a physical problem. Some people can be helped with drugs that dry up saliva production.

Furred or burning tongue

It is common for people who are worried about their health to inspect their tongues in the mirror frequently. Most 'symptoms', such as a 'black furry' tongue, are of no importance. Good mouth hygiene should solve the problem. Possible causes of a furring of the tongue include smoking, fever, mouth-breathing or fasting.

A burning sensation is not usually serious either. It can be caused by ill-fitting dentures or smoking. Sometimes it is caused by a lack of B group vitamins (especially vitamins B_1 and B_{12}), folate and zinc. Most people just need explanation and reassurance.

Lump in the throat

Many people have felt a brief 'lump in the throat', often with a dry mouth, usually during strong emotion, particularly grief – especially if they're trying not to cry. This is quite different from a condition called globus hystericus, which is the sensation of a lump in the throat associated with difficulty in swallowing. This sensation may be brought on by anxiety, especially if it leads to overbreathing (hyperventilation).

Difficulty in swallowing may also be a problem when acid comes up into the oesophagus (called reflux). This often affects people with IBS (see 'Heartburn and related symptoms' below). The difficulty swallowing will usually disappear once the problem of reflux has been treated.

Nausea and vomiting

Nausea and vomiting can result from a wide variety of problems relating to the gut, nervous system and hormone balance. If you also experience abdominal pain and have lost weight, your doctor will probably want to arrange tests to establish the underlying cause.

Nausea on its own, especially if you have been prone to it for some time or experience it repeatedly, is virtually never serious. It is unlikely to mean that you have anything very much wrong with you.

Your doctor may want to discuss possible psychological explanations because nausea and vomiting that occur shortly after a meal are often the result of excessive anxiety. This is especially likely if you have no other symptoms, such as weight loss, and if the results of a barium meal (in which barium is swallowed to outline the oesophagus, stomach and duodenum) and endoscopy tests are normal.

Treatment involves identifying stress factors and helping you to try to deal with them better. Sometimes, you may be given drug treatment to relieve anxiety and to suppress the symptoms.

Heartburn and related symptoms

Around 50 per cent of people with IBS have symptoms of heartburn. This is caused by the partially digested stomach contents flowing back up the oesophagus (refluxing), which can become inflamed as a result. Waterbrash, which is the regurgitation of a clear fluid like saliva into the mouth, is unlikely to be caused by disease. However, your doctor may want you to have tests to rule out a duodenal ulcer as a possible cause. If you have either heartburn or waterbrash, you may be referred to an outpatient clinic for gastroscopy (examination of the oesophagus, stomach and duodenum by inserting an instrument with a camera at its tip).

The gastroscopy examination

A flexible tube is passed down the throat to examine the oesophagus, stomach and duodenum. The gastroscope can cause discomfort, so the patient is offered a throat spray or intravenous sedation. The gastroscope tube has a camera at its tip and the lining of the oesophagus, stomach and duodenum are viewed on a screen.

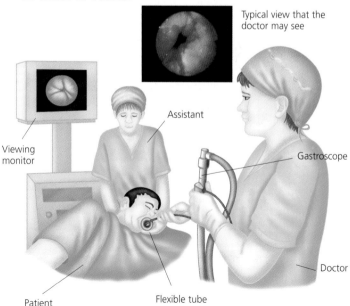

Typical view that the doctor may see

Assistant

Viewing monitor

Gastroscope

Patient

Flexible tube

Doctor

Gastro-oesophageal reflux (heartburn)

Gastro-oesophageal reflux (heartburn) occurs when the acidic stomach contents leak back into the oesophagus, causing the symptoms that we know as heartburn.

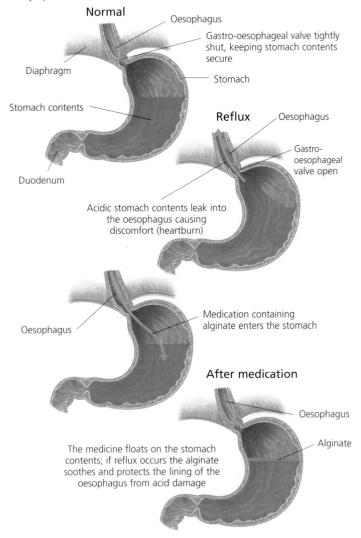

Normal

Oesophagus

Gastro-oesophageal valve tightly shut, keeping stomach contents secure

Diaphragm

Stomach

Stomach contents

Duodenum

Reflux

Oesophagus

Gastro-oesophageal valve open

Acidic stomach contents leak into the oesophagus causing discomfort (heartburn)

Oesophagus

Medication containing alginate enters the stomach

After medication

Oesophagus

Alginate

The medicine floats on the stomach contents; if reflux occurs the alginate soothes and protects the lining of the oesophagus from acid damage

Avoiding heartburn at night

If you lie on a horizontal bed it is easier for your stomach contents to leak into the oesophagus and cause heartburn. Sleeping on a bed raised slightly at the head end can avoid this.

Stomach contents leak into the oesophagus

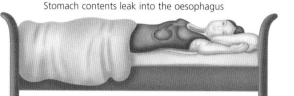

Stomach contents remain in the stomach

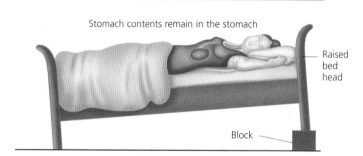

Raised bed head

Block

If you have heartburn, this can usually be treated effectively by simple measures such as losing any excess weight, taking an antacid or acid-blocking drug, and sleeping with the head of your bed raised a few inches (see above).

Feeling uncomfortably full with discomfort around your solar plexus is not usually an indication that anything serious is wrong. However, you will probably be sent for endoscopy of the upper part of your gastrointestinal tract to rule out this possibility. 'Butterflies' in your stomach and a 'sinking feeling in the pit of the abdomen' are unpleasant but rarely symptoms of any serious disorder.

Gas

Many people are both bothered by and mystified by intestinal gas. It is useful to have a few facts about gas (see box opposite).

Excess gas

One of the more interesting statistics about intestinal gas is that healthy people expel intestinal wind (flatus) on average 14 times per day. In fact, it is probable that most people who think that they pass unusually large quantities are not that different in this respect from other people.

Although malabsorption and poor digestion may be responsible for gas production, organic disease is rarely a factor. Often those who are concerned about gas are particularly anxious and may have other emotional problems.

It may be factors such as timing, frequency, noise and smell, rather than total amount passed, that determine whether you perceive gas as a symptom. It can cause problems such as burping, belching, noisy intestinal rumblings (borborygmi), abdominal distension, pain or passing embarrassing amounts of flatus.

How would I know if I have excess gas?

There are two possible ways in which these symptoms can be caused. It may be an increase in the volume of gas in the gastrointestinal tract or it may be a reduction in the rate at which it is expelled or cleared.

An increase in the volume of intestinal gas may result from increased intake of swallowed air or enhanced production of gas in the colon by bacterial fermentation. A reduced rate of clearance of gas is

Facts about gas

We often know little about intestinal gas – and even find it embarrassing. However, it is normal during digestion to produce gas.

Quantity of gas

Normal volume of gas in gastrointestinal tract = 150–200 ml

Normal total volume of gas passed per day = 1,000–1,500 ml

Major components of gas

Oxygen and nitrogen – from swallowed air

Hydrogen – from metabolism of carbohydrates

Methane – a gas that comes from the body's metabolism (how and why it is formed is still unclear: only one person in three has an inherited characteristic that leads to the formation of methane in the intestines)

Smell of gas

The unpleasant smell of gas expelled through the rectum comes from bacterial fermentation of fibre in the colon. This depends on diet – some foods such as onions, garlic and pulses produce more 'smelly' gas than others. The worst smells are of ammonia and sulphur-containing components.

most common in people who have long-term problems of excessive gas, bloating and flatulence.

Some people form a normal amount of intestinal gas but the infusion of gas into their intestines produces more discomfort and pain than normal. This suggests that their symptoms are caused by an abnormal sensitivity of the gut rather than an abnormal stimulus.

Swallowing air

Everyone swallows some air along with saliva when they eat or drink. However, some of those who complain of excess gas in the stomach take in two to three times as much air as fluid.

The habit of swallowing air even when not eating is known as aerophagia. Factors that may encourage it include mouth-breathing, ill-fitting dentures, ulcers or sores in the mouth, smoking, chewing gum, taking certain medications (anticholinergic drugs), bolting your food and emotional disturbance. Some people deliberately swallow air then belch, in an effort to relieve pain caused by angina, oesophageal reflux or other illnesses.

Your doctor will need to find out the reason why you are swallowing air in order to be able to treat the problem properly. One trick that may prove useful in overcoming aerophagy and belching is to place a pen between your teeth. This works because, strictly speaking, the air is not swallowed but sucked into the oesophagus by the negative pressure created when you relax the upper oesophageal sphincter muscle. You can't suck air into your oesophagus with a pen in your mouth!

Bacterial fermentation

Increased production of gas may result from excess bacterial fermentation of carbohydrates in your diet. In healthy people, this normally occurs in the colon. If you have a condition that impairs your digestion or that prevents you absorbing food properly, it may also occur in the small intestine.

If you eat a high-fibre diet, especially one that includes a lot of fruit and vegetables such as pulses and beans, this can result in fermentation. This in turn leads to an increased production of gas, particularly carbon dioxide and hydrogen.

Bacterial fermentation in the colon produces a number of smelly gases such as ammonia and hydrogen sulphide. Although these are present in flatus in only very small quantities, they may be smelt at concentrations as low as one part per million.

Many people resort to eating charcoal biscuits to counteract any tendency to form smelly gas, but there is some doubt about their effectiveness in 'absorbing' intestinal gas. You may help to alleviate your 'gaseous' symptoms by changing your diet, especially reducing the amount of fibre if you normally have a high intake.

Borborygmi

This is the medical term for a noisy, windy, gurgling abdomen. It may be a symptom of malabsorption or poor digestion, but occasionally it may be a sign of some kind of intestinal obstruction. However, when borborygmi is the prime symptom and other diseases have been ruled out, the cause is almost always some kind of functional disturbance.

Proptosis

This is the term for periodic abdominal swelling, often with associated back pain. It affects women more than men. It may develop suddenly, sometimes after food, or it may come on gradually. It can make a woman look pregnant and in both sexes clothes feel tight. The swelling usually subsides within 24 hours.

Proptosis is caused by contraction of the diaphragm and the muscles in the lower back, which compresses the abdominal contents and pushes them forward. Proptosis often accompanies IBS and it is important to recognise that the condition is not caused by organic disease and no further investigation is required.

You don't need treatment either – and your doctor will simply explain why the problem occurs and reassure you that it is nothing to worry about. You may get some relief by lying flat and relaxing your muscles. If you're a very anxious person, your doctor may suggest some kind of treatment to help you relax (see page 96).

Proctalgia fugax

Proctalgia fugax refers to a sudden pain felt deep in the rectum, which may last for a few seconds to several minutes and can vary in intensity. It usually happens at night and is thought to be a symptom of IBS, although it is not one of the standard features of the condition.

It is not serious in itself, and does not necessarily require treatment, although an anti-spasmodic drug may sometimes be prescribed.

Trouble with bowel opening

People with IBS sometimes experience problems to do with opening their bowels. These can include:

- feeling no urge to defecate even though faeces are present in the rectum

- painful involuntary straining (tenesmus)

- ineffectual and painful straining when trying to pass a stool

- the sensation that you can't completely empty your bowels.

Such difficulties are usually functional in origin, but your GP or a hospital doctor will first want to perform a gentle examination of the back passage and sigmoidoscopy, to make sure that they are not caused by any organic disease. You will also have to have tests if you have mucus or runny stools. This is because, although these symptoms occur most commonly in IBS, they can occasionally be caused by inflammatory bowel disease or tumours of the rectum or colon.

KEY POINTS

■ A wide variety of gastrointestinal symptoms and disorders, originating from the mouth to the anus, are associated with IBS

■ Treatment for excessive anxiety can help to alleviate symptoms for many people

■ The intestines of people with IBS are particularly sensitive to gas, which is cleared more slowly than normal from the gut

Treatment

A positive diagnosis can be reassuring

In the past, you would probably have been told you had IBS only when all other possible causes for your symptoms had been ruled out. Today it is diagnosed as a condition in its own right based on the pattern of symptoms.

The fact that any tests have come back negative is very reassuring and confirms that your symptoms are the result of a disorder of bowel function relating to intestinal spasms, gas and/or 'sluggish bowels'. It is also reassuring to know that, although your symptoms may be troublesome, they will produce no complications whatsoever.

It is important to raise any worries you may have such as fear of inflammation, ulceration or cancer so that your doctor can help to put your mind at rest.

Psychological therapies

Many people with IBS also have underlying anxiety which makes their symptoms worse. A number of

What your doctor will do to help you

Once you have been diagnosed with IBS, your doctor will advise you of any changes that you need to make to reduce your symptoms. If there are any treatments that may help, your doctor will suggest these. Help includes the following:

- Reassurance that you do not have a serious illness such as cancer

- Treatment may be needed with bulk laxatives or anti-diarrhoeal or anti-spasmodic drugs

- Treatment may be needed for associated problems such as gynaecological disorders

- Benefit may be obtained from a short course of anti-anxiety or antidepressant drug treatment

psychological therapies can help, although these are not always freely available on the NHS.

Relaxation therapy

This is the simplest form of 'psychotherapy' which you can easily learn from audio tapes. If stress is contributing to your IBS, then relaxation will help to reduce your symptoms and give you a sense of well-being, so that you feel more confident and in control.

You will also be taught how to exclude sources of tension and so relax. Usually, around 10 sessions are needed.

Biofeedback

This depends on recognising various signs of abnormal body function and learning how to correct them. It is most commonly used in the treatment of incontinence and constipation.

Therapy aims to make you more sensitive to rectal sensation and avoid inappropriate straining. It also provides a detailed explanation of how your body normally works, and helps to retrain your bowel actions.

Hypnotherapy

Hypnosis is used to induce a state of relaxation and then to try to alter underlying abnormalities of gut motility and/or sensation.

The therapist will hypnotise you, with the ultimate aim of enabling you to control symptoms on your own, by making use of what you have learned during the treatment sessions. Success depends very much on the therapist being interested in treating IBS.

Cognitive–behavioural therapy

Cognitive–behavioural therapy (CBT) is based on the assumption that IBS in some people is related to the way that you respond to what happens in your everyday life. CBT helps you to recognise negative patterns of thinking and behaviour.

It encourages you to change your interpretation of bodily sensations and functions by seeing them differently. It helps if you see them not so much as symptoms of disease that need to be treated, but more as expressions of anxiety that are associated with particular life events. Treatment is essentially an exercise in identifying and solving problems, which allows you to gain a greater sense of control.

Dynamic psychotherapy

This helps to provide you with an insight into why

particular symptoms have developed and what they might mean or represent in the light of changes in key relationships. These insights will help you make long-lasting changes in your normal attitudes and behaviour patterns.

Symptoms often seem to stem from significant life changes (often the loss of a relationship) that are difficult to come to terms with. This therapy helps you work through relationship difficulties with the guidance of the therapist.

How effective are psychological therapies?

Most studies with behavioural therapy, psychotherapy or hypnotherapy show that brief treatments result in a 60 to 70 per cent improvement in IBS symptoms. Young people who have had classic symptoms for a relatively short time do best. However, 15–20 per cent of people with IBS do not benefit at all from psychological therapies.

Drug treatment

Unfortunately, drug treatments for IBS are of only limited value and many have side effects. Nevertheless, some drugs may help certain symptoms in individual people.

It may be that you need only one drug, although some people do better on a combination of drugs. An example is a laxative or anti-diarrhoeal drug (see page 75) together with a drug that reduces muscle spasm or anxiety. A combination of an anti-anxiety drug and an antidepressant can relieve abdominal pain and diarrhoea effectively for some people.

Combining drugs in this way may make it possible to control your condition with smaller doses than when one is prescribed on its own. However, there is also a greater risk of side effects.

Anti-spasmodic drugs

Anti-spasmodic drugs (such as mebeverine, dicyclomine, alverine citrate and hyoscine butylbromide) relax intestinal smooth muscle. They may be helpful in relieving pain caused by spasms of the colon. Some people find that these drugs stop working after a while, but it is usually possible for your doctor to prescribe a related drug if

Anti-spasmodic drugs

If you suffer from pain caused by strong spasms in your colon, anti-spasmodic drugs may help. They act by relaxing the intestinal muscles.

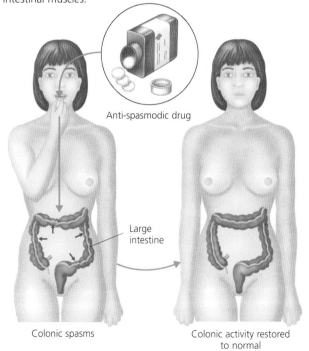

Anti-spasmodic drug

Large
intestine

Colonic spasms

Colonic activity restored
to normal

this happens. This is likely to remain effective for a similar period of time to the first drug.

Some people benefit from having hyoscine (see above) injected just under the skin or into a muscle. If you experience severe functional pain that comes on suddenly, you (or a member of your family or a carer) can be taught to give an injection at the first sign of an attack.

Antidepressant drugs

As well as treating underlying depression, antidepressants can change the way that your gut muscles react and alter nerve responses from your gut. One such drug, called imipramine, slows down the rapid small bowel transit, which is the problem for people with diarrhoea-predominant IBS. Another drug, called paroxetine (a selective serotonin reuptake inhibitor or SSRI), accelerates movement of the contents through the small bowel.

Both these treatments can relieve gut symptoms at doses too low to have any effect on your state of mind. Antidepressant medication has also been shown to have significant benefit in the treatment of pain. These drugs are most effective when taken at night.

Other antidepressants affect the response to serotonin. Serotonin (also known as hydroxytryptamine) is a hormone with an important role in the motor (movement) and secretory response of the gut to the ingestion of food. One of these drugs is alosetron which antagonises type 3 serotonin (HT_3) receptors in the gut and is effective in diarrhoea-predominant IBS, although vascular damage to the colon has been linked to its use.

Another is tegaserod, which stimulates type 4 serotonin (HT_4) receptors. It is now available in the USA and some other countries, but not in the UK, for constipation-predominant IBS in women.

Dietary treatment

If your diet is contributing to your symptoms, making changes can bring considerable relief. This could be something as simple as reducing your intake of natural fibre foods, fruit or caffeine, if any are on the high side.

Some people, especially those of non-European descent, may not produce enough of the lactase enzyme (needed to digest the milk sugar, lactose). If you regularly consume more than half a pint (280 millilitres) of milk a day, you may benefit from cutting down.

A few people develop IBS symptoms from a high intake of fructose (fruit sugar) as a result of slow or incomplete absorption. It can cause gut distension to which people with IBS appear to be especially sensitive.

You may have already identified for yourself certain foods that trigger your symptoms, especially if you are prone to diarrhoea. If this leads you to limit the range of foods that you eat, you should ask your doctor to refer you to a dietitian to make sure that you continue to obtain all the nutrients that you need from your restricted diet.

Aloe vera is a herbal remedy that has been used medically for thousands of years. Some people claim that it has helped their symptoms of IBS. Others, however, have reported that their symptoms have got worse. In the absence of properly conducted clinical trials showing any benefit, its routine use cannot be recommended

Similarly, scientific evidence to support the use of Yakult, avoiding yeast-containing food and drink or following a gluten-free diet in IBS is also lacking. Yakult is a fermented milk drink that contains lactobacilli. These promote the growth of friendly bacteria in the gut and inhibit the overgrowth of potentially harmful ones. When tested, however, lactobacilli did not improve IBS symptoms (but see below).

Avoidance of yeast-containing foods has been suggested in the belief that this will prevent candidiasis (overgrowth of the candida organism – a kind of yeast) in the gut. However, scientific evidence suggests that *Candida* is not involved in causing IBS.

A small minority of people find that excluding gluten (contained in wheat, barley and rye) from their diet helps their IBS, but most stay the same or actually get worse.

Complementary and alternative therapies

A wide variety of complementary and alternative practices and therapies is commonly used by IBS patients, both together with and instead of conventional treatment. As many of these therapies have not been subjected to controlled clinical trials, some at least of their efficacy may reflect the high placebo response rate seen in IBS.

There is, however, evidence to support the efficacy in IBS for hypnotherapy, some forms of herbal therapy and certain probiotics.

Probiotics are 'friendly bacteria', such as lactobacilli and bifidobacteria. They have several actions that may be of benefit in IBS. These include antibacterial effects, protection of the gut lining and influencing immune reactions in the gut.

When treatment doesn't help

Around five per cent of people continue to experience abdominal pain that causes a major disturbance to their lives, despite having tried all the standard treatments. This can be frustrating for both the doctor and the person affected, especially when investigations repeatedly find no cause for the problem.

It might seem logical for the person to be referred to a specialist (or even more than one) and particularly to a psychiatrist. However, in practice this often doesn't help and can just make existing anxiety worse.

A more successful approach may be for you to continue to see the same doctor (either your GP or an individual hospital doctor) every few months or so to review the situation and discuss your current symptoms. Eventually, this may help you to come to terms with your affliction and enhance your ability to cope with it.

KEY POINTS

■ The diagnosis of IBS is a positive one, and is not based simply on ruling out any other possible causes for your symptoms

■ Don't be upset if your doctor suggests that psychological problems may have a role in causing your symptoms, as this is often the case

■ Psychological therapies, including relaxation therapy, biofeedback, hypnotherapy and psychotherapy, are often helpful

■ Drug treatments for IBS are of limited value, but may help to relieve individual symptoms, especially abdominal pain

■ Sometimes a change in your diet may relieve symptoms if this is playing a part in triggering your symptoms

What happens now?

Living with IBS

If you have been referred to a hospital specialist, whether you need further appointments and, if so, how frequently will depend on your personal situation. You may well have found that you have been given a satisfactory explanation for your symptoms and don't need to see the doctor again, especially if your IBS is no more than a minor inconvenience.

You may need to have follow-up appointments if you have been advised to alter your intake of fibre and/or if you have been put on medication. This is so that your response to treatment can be assessed, and the visits may continue until such time as your symptoms have stabilised or until it seems that you are unlikely to benefit further by continuing to attend the clinic.

However, it is important that you have a good line of communication with either your GP or the clinic doctor so that you feel that you can return if you need to. Some people will need to continue seeing their doctor on a regular basis, to monitor the situation and discuss symptoms and worries.

If you think that your GP is unsympathetic and you cannot establish a good relationship, you might ask whether another doctor in the practice has a particular interest in IBS.

Outlook

Unfortunately, once you have IBS, you are likely to continue having symptoms and, although they may come and go, a permanent cure is unlikely. The most striking feature is that symptoms tend to remain constant, although the severity will vary from time to time.

A substantial proportion of individuals with IBS become free from symptoms over a 12-month period, but may develop other functional symptoms such as indigestion (dyspepsia) in their place. In one study, around 30 per cent of people with IBS still had symptoms after five years. Another study found that only five per cent of people were completely symptom free after five years.

You are likely to have a less optimistic outlook in terms of getting rid of your symptoms if:

- psychological factors (such as anxiety) have a major role in causing them
- you have had IBS for a long time
- you have had abdominal surgery.

Most people learn to live with their problem and find that explanation and reassurance from their doctor are the most important aspect of their treatment. You should always let your doctor know if your symptoms change significantly. However, once the diagnosis of IBS is established, the chances of developing some new and serious disease are extremely low.

KEY POINTS

- IBS is a long-term problem, although symptoms may come and go, but a permanent cure is unlikely

- Whether you need to have follow-up appointments once your condition has been diagnosed will depend on individual circumstances

- Most people can learn to live with their IBS symptoms which, although they can be troublesome, are very unlikely to lead to any complications

- If you have IBS, your chances of remaining free of serious disease are excellent

Useful addresses

We have included the following organisations because, on preliminary investigation, they may be of use to the reader. However, we do not have first-hand experience of each organisation and so cannot guarantee the organisation's integrity. The reader must therefore exercise his or her own discretion and judgement when making further enquiries.

Benefits Enquiry Line
Tel: 0800 882200
Minicom: 0800 243355
Website: www.dwp.gov.uk
N. Ireland: 0800 220674

Government agency giving information and advice on sickness and disability benefits for people with disabilities and their carers.

Citizens Advice Bureaux
Myddleton House, 115–123 Pentonville Road
London N1 9LZ

Tel: 020 7833 2181 (admin only)
Website: www.adviceguide.org.uk

HQ of national charity offering a wide variety of practical, financial and legal advice. Network of local charities throughout the UK listed in phone books and in *Yellow Pages* under 'C'.

Continence Foundation
307 Hatton Square, 16 Baldwins Gardens
London EC1N 7RJ
Tel: 020 7404 6875
Fax: 020 7404 6876
Helpline: 0845 345 0165 (Mon–Fri 9.30am–1pm)
Email: continence.foundation@dial.pipex.com
Website: www.continence-foundation.org.uk

Offers information and support for people with bladder and/or bowel problems. Has list of regional specialists. An SAE requested.

CORE (Digestive Disorders Foundation)
3 St Andrew's Place, Regents Park
London NW1 4LB
Tel: 020 7486 0341
Fax: 020 7224 2012
Email: info@corecharity.org.uk
Website: www.digestivedisorders.org.uk

Provides a range of leaflets about the cause, symptoms and treatment of digestive disorders on receipt of an SAE. Medical advice not available over the phone.

IBS Network – The Irritable Bowel Syndrome Network
Unit 5, Mowbray Street
Sheffield S3 8EN
Tel: 0114 272 3253 (Mon–Fri 6pm–8pm, Sat 10am–12 noon)
Fax: 0114 261 0112
Email: info@ibsnetwork.org.uk
Website: www.ibsnetwork.org.uk

Publishes factsheets and quarterly newsletter and coordinates local self-help groups, which offer a befriending scheme giving support to fellow sufferers. Helpline staffed by IBS nurse specialists. An SAE required for information by post.

IBS Self Help Group (Irritable Bowel Syndrome Association)
1440 Whalley Avenue, No. 145, New Haven
CT 06515, USA
Email: ibsa@ibsassociation.org
Website: www.ibsassociation.org

USA-based international website with information and online forum; provides access to bulletin and chat boards, book list and store, medication (available in North America) and clinical study listings. No implied endorsement of sponsored products advertised; all donations fund activities of the Group.

Incontact – Action on Incontinence
United House, North Road
London N7 9DP
Tel: 0870 770 3246

Fax: 0870 770 3249
Email: info@incontact.org
Website: www.incontact.org

Information and help via local support and user groups
for people with bladder and bowel problems and their
carers. Has list of suppliers of incontinence pads.

National Institute for Health and Clinical Excellence (NICE)

MidCity Place, 71 High Holborn
London WC1V 6NA
Tel: 020 7067 5800
Fax: 020 7067 5801
Email: nice@nice.nhs.uk
Website: www.nice.org.uk

Provides national guidance on the promotion of good
health and the prevention and treatment of ill-health.
Patient information leaflets are available for each piece
of guidance issued.

NHS Direct

Tel: 0845 4647 (24 hours, 365 days a year)
Textphone 0845 606 4647
Website: www.nhsdirect.nhs.uk
NHS Scotland: 0800 224488

Offers confidential health-care advice, information and
referral service. A good first port of call for any health
advice.

NHS Smoking Helplines

Tel: 0800 169 0169 (7am–11pm, 365 days a year)

Pregnancy smoking helpline: 0800 169 9169
(12noon–9pm, 365 days a year)
Website: www.givingupsmoking.co.uk

Have advice, help and encouragement on giving up
smoking. Specialist advisers available to offer on-going
support to those who genuinely are trying to give up
smoking. Can refer to local branches.

Prodigy Website
Sowerby Centre for Health Informatics at Newcastle
(SCHIN), Bede House, All Saints Business Centre
Newcastle upon Tyne NE1 2ES
Tel: 0191 243 6100
Fax: 0191 243 6101
Email: prodigy-enquiries@schin.co.uk
Website: www.prodigy.nhs.uk

A website mainly for GPs giving information for
patients listed by disease plus named self-help
organisations.

Quit (Smoking Quitlines)
211 Old Street
London EC1V 9NR
Helpline: 0800 002 200 (9am–9pm, 365 days a year)
Tel: 020 7251 1551
Fax: 020 7251 1661
Email: info@quit.org.uk
Website: www.quit.org.uk
Scotland: 0800 848484
Wales: 0800 169 0169 (NHS)

Offers individual advice on giving up smoking in English and Asian languages. Talks to schools on smoking and pregnancy and can refer to local support groups. Runs training courses for professionals.

UK Register of IBS Hypnotherapists
PO Box 57
Warrington WA5 1FG
Tel: 0800 085 3970
Website: www.ibs-register.co.uk

Website offering lists of UK hypnotherapists specialising in IBS. It is a 'commercial' site, owned by one of the practitioners who advises patients to check all qualifications before treatment. Also produces self-help hypnotherapy CDs.

The internet as a source of further information

After reading this book, you may feel that you would like further information on the subject. The internet is of course an excellent place to look and there are many websites with useful information about medical disorders, related charities and support groups.

For those who do not have a computer at home some bars and cafes offer facilities for accessing the internet. These are listed in the *Yellow Pages* under 'Internet Bars and Cafes' and 'Internet Providers'. Your local library offers a similar facility and has staff to help you find the information that you need.

It should always be remembered, however, that the internet is unregulated and anyone is free to set up a website and add information to it. Many websites offer impartial advice and information that has been compiled and checked by qualified medical professionals. Some, on the other hand, are run by commercial organisations with the purpose of promoting their own products. Others still are run by pressure groups, some of which will provide carefully assessed and accurate information whereas others may be suggesting medications or treatments that are not supported by the medical and scientific community.

Unless you know the address of the website you want to visit – for example, www.familydoctor.co.uk – you may find the following guidelines useful when searching the internet for information.

Search engines and other searchable sites

Google (www.google.co.uk) is the most popular search engine used in the UK, followed by Yahoo! (http://uk.yahoo.com) and MSN (www.msn.co.uk). Also popular are the search engines provided by Internet Service Providers such as Tiscali and other sites such as the BBC site (www.bbc.co.uk).

In addition to the search engines that index the whole web, there are also medical sites with search facilities, which act almost like mini-search engines, but cover only medical topics or even a particular area of medicine. Again, it is wise to look at who is responsible for compiling the information offered to ensure that it is impartial and medically accurate. The NHS Direct site (www.nhsdirect.nhs.uk) is an example of a searchable medical site.

Links to many British medical charities can be found at the Association of Medical Research Charities' website (www.amrc.org.uk) and at Charity Choice (www.charitychoice.co.uk).

Search phrases

Be specific when entering a search phrase. Searching for information on 'cancer' will return results for many different types of cancer as well as on cancer in general. You may even find sites offering astrological information. More useful results will be returned by using search phrases such as 'lung cancer' and 'treatments for lung cancer'. Both Google and Yahoo! offer an advanced search option that includes the ability to search for the exact phrase; enclosing the search phrase in quotes, that is, 'treatments for lung cancer', will have the same effect. Limiting a search to an exact phrase reduces the number of results returned but it is best to refine a search to an exact match only if you are not getting useful results with a normal search. Adding 'UK' to your search term will bring up mainly British sites, so a good phrase might be 'lung cancer' UK (don't include UK within the quotes).

Always remember the internet is international and unregulated. It holds a wealth of valuable information but individual sites may be biased, out of date or just plain wrong. Family Doctor Publications accepts no responsibility for the content of links published in this series.

Index

Your pages

We have included the following pages because they may help you manage your illness or condition and its treatment.

Before an appointment with a health professional, it can be useful to write down a short list of questions of things that you do not understand, so that you can make sure that you do not forget anything.

Some of the sections may not be relevant to your circumstances.

We are always pleased to receive constructive criticism or suggestions about how to improve the books. You can contact us at:

Email: familydoctor@btinternet.com
Letter: Family Doctor Publications
        PO Box 4664
        Poole
        BH15 1NN

Thank you

Health-care contact details

Name:

Job title:

Place of work:

Tel:

Name:

Job title:

Place of work:

Tel:

Name:

Job title:

Place of work:

Tel:

Name:

Job title:

Place of work:

Tel:

Significant past health events – illnesses/operations/investigations/treatments

Event	Month	Year	Age (at time)

Appointments for health care

Name:

Place:

Date:

Time:

Tel:

Name:

Place:

Date:

Time:

Tel:

Name:

Place:

Date:

Time:

Tel:

Name:

Place:

Date:

Time:

Tel:

Appointments for health care

Name:

Place:

Date:

Time:

Tel:

Name:

Place:

Date:

Time:

Tel:

Name:

Place:

Date:

Time:

Tel:

Name:

Place:

Date:

Time:

Tel:

Current medication(s) prescribed by your doctor

Medicine name:

Purpose:

Frequency & dose:

Start date:

End date:

Medicine name:

Purpose:

Frequency & dose:

Start date:

End date:

Medicine name:

Purpose:

Frequency & dose:

Start date:

End date:

Medicine name:

Purpose:

Frequency & dose:

Start date:

End date:

Other medicines/supplements you are taking, not prescribed by your doctor

Medicine/treatment:

Purpose:

Frequency & dose:

Start date:

End date:

Medicine/treatment:

Purpose:

Frequency & dose:

Start date:

End date:

Medicine/treatment:

Purpose:

Frequency & dose:

Start date:

End date:

Medicine/treatment:

Purpose:

Frequency & dose:

Start date:

End date:

Questions to ask at appointments

(Note: do bear in mind that doctors work under great time pressure, so long lists may not be helpful for either of you)

Questions to ask at appointments
(Note: do bear in mind that doctors work under great time pressure, so long lists may not be helpful for either of you)

Notes

Notes

Notes

Notes

Notes